★ ★ ★ ★ ★ Teri Tom, MS, RD ★ ★ ★ ★ ★

MARTIAL ARTS NUTRITION

A PRECISION GUIDE TO FUELING YOUR FIGHTING EDGE

TUTTLE PUBLISHING
Tokyo • Rutland, Vermont • Singapore

Published by Tuttle Publishing, an imprint of Periplus Editions (HK) Ltd., with editorial offices at 364 Innovation Drive, North Clarendon, Vermont 05759 U.S.A. and at 61 Tai Seng Avenue #02-12, Singapore 534167.

Library of Congress Cataloging-in-Publication Data

Tom, Teri.
  Martial arts nutrition : a precision guide to fueling your fighting edge / Teri Tom.
      p. cm.
  Includes bibliographical references and index.
  ISBN 978-0-8048-3931-0 (pbk. : alk. paper)
 1. Nutrition. 2. Martial artists--Nutrition. 3. Exercise--Physiological aspects. I. Title.
  RA784.T645 2009
  613.7'148--dc22   2009013674

ISBN 978-0-8048-3931-0

Distributed by

North America, Latin America & Europe
Tuttle Publishing
364 Innovation Drive
North Clarendon, VT 05759-9436 U.S.A.
Tel: 1 (802) 773-8930; Fax: 1 (802) 773-6993
info@tuttlepublishing.com; www.tuttlepublishing.com

Asia Pacific
Berkeley Books Pte. Ltd.
61 Tai Seng Avenue #02-12
Singapore 534167
Tel: (65) 6280-1330; Fax: (65) 6280-6290
inquiries@periplus.com.sg; www.periplus.com

First edition
12 11 10 09   5 4 3 2 1

Printed in Singapore

TUTTLE PUBLISHING® is a registered trademark of Tuttle Publishing, a division of Periplus Editions (HK) Ltd.

Contents

To Katherine Lee Tom and Hohn D. Tom

ACKNOWLEDGMENTS

Special thanks to:

Rosie Flores for questioning my diet
Lucho Crisalle for the mentoring and WhatWorks® software
New Leaf
Sensei Peter Freedman
Brett Benson
Andrei Arlovski
Amir Khan
Manny Pacquiao
Freddie Roach and Wildcard Boxing Club
My clients at the Sports Club/LA
The Crew for not letting my blood sugar dip too low
Sandra Korinchak, my editor at Tuttle

And extra special thanks to Alex Ariza for taking a chance.

The Surefire Way to a Better Body

By the time most of my clients come to me, they've already tried just about every diet under the sun. They've done no carbs, all grapefruit, cabbage soup, and nasty cayenne pepper concoctions. Some of them have exercised themselves into the ground but didn't watch their diets. Others dieted themselves into a frenzy but didn't budge from the couch, while others did both—exercised and dieted like maniacs—and still didn't see any progress. And some clients had gotten just plain bad advice. I've seen these pitfalls on every level, from weekend warriors to the elite levels of the UFC and WBC.

My point, and the approach you'll be benefiting from throughout this book, is that to reach your fitness goals, you need to have all the variables in place. Haphazardly throwing together elements of a fitness program might get you some results, but when you hit a plateau, you won't know how to break through it. This is why I hate the general guidelines that most nutrition books offer. Yes, you should eat healthy fats, but how much? Too much of anything—even flax seed oil—gets stored as fat. Yes, you should exercise, but if you feel like you're gonna yak, then you're pushing too hard and burning muscle, not fat. Yes, you need to eat six times a day, but at what times, and how much, and in what ratios?

If there's one thing I've learned from seeing hundreds of clients over the years, it's that everyone is different. Everyone has a unique response to both food and exercise. There's no one-size-fits-all cookie-cutter approach that works. So what I'll do here is give you the tools necessary to cover all your bases. I'll provide methods for determining your specific caloric needs, equations to determine the intensity of your workouts, templates for meal planning, and, most important, the steps you'll need to take based on your week-to-week results.

I tell clients that I'm essentially running a scientific procedure on them from week to week. We cover exercise variables of frequency, duration, and intensity. We also control for nutrition variables—meal times, amounts (calories), and ratios (of protein, carbs, and fat). With all those bases covered we are solving for one variable: your body composition. This is the piece of information that tells me if any dietary changes are necessary and if so, what they are and how to go about making those changes.

New clients are always surprised by this scientific approach. "Wow," they say, "I had no idea that there was this much to it." Well, there really isn't. Fitness is a science, but it's not rocket science. With all the proper variables in place, there is *no* reason why you shouldn't be able to reach your goals, because you will no longer be shooting in the dark. And even if you already are seeing results from generalized guidelines, you'll hit your goals a lot faster if you become more precise about controlling for the variables. So when you do hit a plateau—and everyone does eventually—you'll know exactly what's been going on and whether you have to turn left or right to get to the next level.

The funny thing is that many clients tell me that my methods are "secret" solutions they've never heard before, but truthfully, I'm sure you've heard of them all at one time or another. The difference is that I've organized them for you in one comprehensive, scientific package. They work best only if *all* the puzzle pieces are in place. Any one of these elements alone—even exercise—is not going to get you optimal results.

This includes, by the way, one very important component—your head. What's going on upstairs is vital to your success. All the science in the world isn't going to help if you aren't clear about what's setting you into action.

With the proper motivation and tools behind you, you *cannot* fail with this method. And since this book is geared toward the martial arts and combat sports, most of you reading this know how important it is not to have any weak links in your fighting arsenal. The same principle applies to your approach to nutrition and fitness. Train and fuel yourself methodically, and you can't miss on this plan.

CHAPTER 1

My Story, and What It Means for You

The road to the creation of this book has been a strangely circuitous one. From my nutrition practice at The Sports Club/LA to my clientele at Wildcard Boxing Club, people always ask me how I got into "the field." It wasn't a choice, I tell them. It was an act of survival. I share it here to give you some insight into the development of my approach.

When I was at UCLA, eating well was not exactly at the top of my list. Outside of school, I was playing surfabilly guitar in smoky clubs all over LA and the West Coast. My band had just started to generate some major label interest and had been invited to play overseas. Even more important, I had the opportunity to play alongside and learn from some of my music heroes.

I should have been having the time of my life, but I wasn't. I could barely breathe. Playing in smoky clubs four nights a week had wreaked havoc on my lungs. And being in a band—well, let's just say we didn't eat and we didn't sleep. We played all night, worked during the day, went to the next gig, played all night, worked, drove to the gig, played all night… You get the idea.

The combination of the two trashed my immune system. If someone with a bug looked at me I'd get it. This would turn into a respiratory infection, which would, in turn, trigger an asthmatic spell that could last for weeks. It would always devolve into bronchial spasms that persisted all day and worsened at night. Unable to take a single normal breath without coughing it back out, I was kept awake by retching fits for weeks at a time.

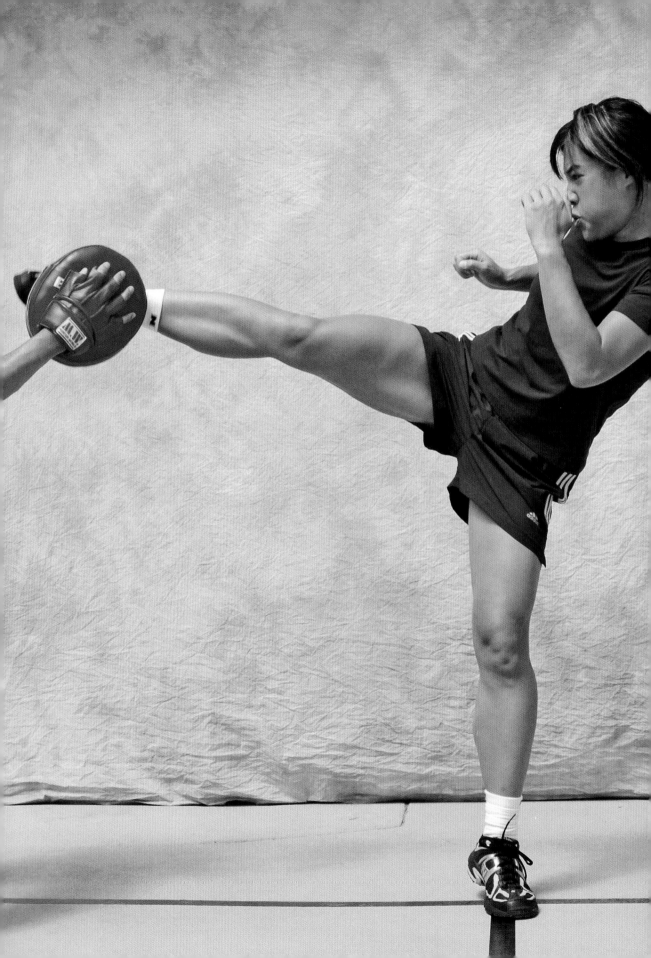

Initially, the doctors misdiagnosed me with bronchitis and gave me antibiotics. But this didn't solve the coughing problem. It just made me more susceptible to infection. After almost two years, they finally entertained the possibility that it might be asthma. So they would give me both antibiotics *and* anti-inflammatories to knock out the asthmatic attacks. In the short term, this worked. But I was getting respiratory infections—sinus infections, chest colds, you name it—with much greater frequency, just about every other week. This meant even more antibiotics and anti–inflammatories, a weakened immune system, more antibiotics and anti–inflammatories, a further weakened immune system, and the downward spiral continued.

I was only a few years out of college, but I was sure I would never see 30. And I probably wouldn't have except for the suggestion of a good friend. After hearing me hack away in the studio from 4:30 in the afternoon to 6:00 in the morning, unable to take a single normal breath, this friend said with typical understatement, "You don't sound too good. Maybe you should try changing your diet."

DIET?! What diet? We don't eat! We don't sleep! Come to think of it, my band mates weren't exactly pictures of health either. We'd just pass bugs around. From the bass player, to the singer, to the drummer. From the drummer, to the bass player, to the singer. From the singer, to the drummer, to the bass player. And me, I *always* had the bug *du jour*.

So when my friend in the studio suggested changing up eating habits, at that time, I would've tried anything. The doctors weren't helping. Medication wasn't helping. As a kid, I'd played a lot of competitive sports—soccer, basketball, softball, volleyball, tennis, track. At UCLA, I'd been running six miles a day. I was now nearly incapacitated, barely able to get off the couch, and completely incapable of breathing. Getting out the front door was a major event. What did I have to lose by changing my diet?

The next day I got some books on nutrition. They weren't anything outlandish—just good sound advice. I finished the books that day, hobbled out to the supermarket, and started following the guidelines.

This is the crazy part. In three weeks, hmm, I felt pretty good. I was off the couch and walking around. In three months, I was like a new person. At that point, physically, I felt good. But I was angry. How can you graduate Phi Beta Kappa and *summa cum laude* and not know how to feed yourself? Why don't

The author, post rock 'n' roll days.

they teach this stuff in school? Why don't they teach it in *elementary* schools? So I decided to get my masters degree in nutritional science and learn how to do this thing the right way. And when I got out maybe I'd save a few people the trouble of going through the same ordeal I had.

It took six years to realize this goal, but it's easily the single best decision I ever made. Every organic chemistry exam, every bio-chem lab, every hour of my clinical rotation at Cedars-Sinai was worth it.

Every day people come into my office frustrated, lacking energy, not feeling well, not seeing results, and not knowing what to do. Their doctors are threatening them with cholesterol medication, alarming lab results, and diagnoses of diabetes and hypertension. After a few weeks of following their individualized plans, the changes they see are amazing—and incredibly rewarding. You'll read the success stories from just a few of my clients later in this book. I've also included their progress charts so you can see how we got them to where they are now. This will give you a glimpse of what is possible for you.

Of course, I also have my share of clients who are already well on their way to healthy lifestyles and are only seeking fine-tuning in either body composition or athletic performance. You'll find guidelines for these goals as well. The basic principles remain the same. Only minor tweaks are required to customize a plan and tailor it to the individual.

Because this is a book geared toward peak performance in the martial arts and sport, it only makes sense to follow the lead of those quintessential warriors, the samurai, in our approach to health and fitness. Their incorporation of Zen Buddhism into daily life provides the perfect roadmap to guide us through this journey toward self-actualization.

Over the years, I've come to recognize particular patterns of success. I've whittled them down to 10 principles. They are *not* the only elements of success, but they do have to be in place for real, lasting results. Nor are they exclusive to Zen or Asian culture; you will find similar themes in areas from pop psychology to the Transcendentalists. I use this Zen framework, though, because of my martial arts background and because this book—while its principles apply to everyone, regardless of their athletic endeavors—is geared toward athletes, particularly those in combat sports.

I've shared my story with you here in the hopes of demonstrating that change is within reach. It is possible to go from a near-complete inability to breathe to being able to spar a full 12 rounds. From being virtually bedridden to sprinting up a hill with your heart rate at 104% of what's estimated as the *maximum* heart rate for your age group. It's possible to put on 20 pounds of muscle. It's possible to improve your VO$_2$ max. It is possible to completely re-build your body.

Again, some of you may only be fine-tuning, eking out that last pound or two of body fat, or trying to put on a few more pounds of muscle. But I also know that some of you are coming from the same place I did. You feel like you're down for the count and reversing that downward momentum seems impossible. If you are ready to receive the information here, though—if you can accept it with Beginner's Mind and persist on a consistent basis—then I guarantee you that momentum will start to shift in your favor. Let's begin.

CHAPTER 2

Lessons from the Battlefield

"This manifold universe functions according to love, but all the shapes and forms we see are in fact just aspects of the one. All the different aspects of human nature, too, are universal manifestations of love. Be aware of these principles when you act, even in such mundane, everyday acts as eating. Food is a gift from the universe. No, in a sense food is the universe."

—Morihei Ueshiba[1]

This book is about fueling yourself properly so that you may engage in combat sports—fighting. In the modern age, we tend to forget the very real life-and-death origins of our chosen martial disciplines. For the general population, the connection between how we treat our bodies and our very survival is much subtler now, but it's still there. And for fighters, that cause-and-effect relationship is more direct and urgent.

To stay fighting fit over the long haul, then, it's helpful to take some cues from the mindset of the samurai, for whom any edge over their opponents could mean the difference between life and death. For you fighters, this should always be at the forefront of your thinking. Combat sports are nothing to play around with, and while they may be sports and they may be fun, they are still dangerous.

For non-combatants reading this book, just remember your body is changing with every second. At any given moment, you are doing something either to delay or accelerate the decline of your body. Do not neglect the seemingly mundane aspects of everyday life, for they add up to something big, namely your health.

How you treat your body day in and day out can determine or prevent a life-or-death situation. To understand this life-and-death mindset, then, we'll be delving into some of the tenets of Zen Buddhism.

It may seem somewhat incongruous—pairing the compassion of Zen with the brutality of the samurai—but the simplicity and clarity of Zen had great appeal to the samurai. It provided a means of self-expression and an approach to training, and gave meaning to that training.

If you are reading this book just for your general health, the samurai approach to Zen can help bring the relationship between your fitness and mortality to the forefront of your awareness. And if you are engaged in combat sports or the martial arts, this mindset and the information in this book can go a long way toward ensuring your safety, optimal performance, and longevity.

Beginner's Mind

In Zen philosophy, beginners of any discipline are said to begin at the stage of Ignorance and Affects. In the study of the sword, for instance, movement is instinctual and natural at this stage because beginners have no point of reference. As they continue training, they become hindered by the conscious effort required to learn a new technique. Conscious thought taints the purity of their actions. According to Takuan Soho, author of one of the great Zen writings, *The Unfettered Mind,* such self-consciousness causes your mind to "stop," preventing you from performing at your best. But after years of technical refinement, an expert is able to perform at the highest skill level without the hindrance of conscious thought, a state that Takuan called *mushin*. He merely acts. And so the circle is complete. The Beginner's Mind is now paired with the expert's skill level.[2] But to get there, you must first be ready to receive instruction.

Before we can start formulating your nutrition plan, you need to be receptive to the information we'll be presenting. Sometimes potential clients will come in and ask about what I do, but they are clearly not ready to let go of their preconceived notions. And it's no wonder with all the information and *mis*information out there. Most of these potential clients are hanging on to the commonly held beliefs that eating less and exercising harder are the answers. Clearly this isn't always the case, though, or they wouldn't be turning up at my office door. And yet, some people come to me expecting to do the same thing they've always done or some variation of it. As soon as I sense this kind of resistance, I usually send them home and tell them to return if/when they are ready to try something different. After all, the definition of insanity is doing the same thing over and over expecting different results.

Other crazy notions for losing body fat include cutting out all starch/breads, eating once a day, slurping only cabbage soup, doing cardio at the expense of resistance training, exercising on an empty stomach, starvation, and the biggest offender of all: using weight as a marker of progress. Now, I'm all about results. My motto is, "If we're gettin' away with it, then keep doing it." But if you're not seeing results, why would you hang on to methods that are clearly not working for you? And yet I've had clients resist me every step of the way, even when we were seeing results!

You'll want to leave any emotional baggage at the door, too. Some clients have mental blocks against certain weight plateaus (again, not my choice of progress marker), clothes sizes, or exercise performance limits. Sometimes a client thinks that because he's never broken the 200-pound mark, he won't be able to do it this time around. And with thinking like that, he won't.

By the way, resistance occurs at all levels—from my casually active clients to the professional fighters. The ones who succeed, of course, are the ones who are eventually willing to empty their knowledge cups.

The Stage of Artlessness

Continuing with our thread of Beginner's Mind is the distinction between the Stage of Art and the Stage of Artlessness. In congruence with Zen teachings, Bruce Lee identified three stages of learning, or "cultivation," as he called it. They are the Stage of Innocence, the Stage of Art, and the Stage of Artlessness.[3] The Stage of Innocence is, of course, the Beginner's Mind, the start of our journey. The Stage of Art is where we consciously learn the skills and master the information of our chosen discipline. And the Stage of Artlessness occurs when we have mastered the skills of our discipline to such a degree that we no longer have to consciously think about them. We just do.

Most of this book is comprised of the Stage of Art. I will give you the information you need to formulate and implement a nutrition plan based on your individual fitness goals. I will also give you a fair amount of background information to explain *why* the plans are constructed as they are. It's important for you to know the scientific basis behind your actions. The bulk of this volume dwells on the Stage of Art because there is a certain amount of material you will need to master and a number of variables you will have to control for in order for the plan to work.

A portion of this book consists of some client case studies. I say that these clients have reached the Stage of Artlessness, because they have mastered the principles of their eating and exercise plans to the extent that they no longer have to think about them. Their plans have become a way of life. Some clients are initially intimidated by the numbers and spreadsheets I use to formulate their plans and chart their progress. They soon come to realize, though, that the precision actually enables them to think *less*. Prior to coming to me, they acknowledge that they used to waste a lot of time and mental energy trying to figure out if they ate too much, ate too little, didn't exercise enough, didn't eat on time, had to make up for the meal or exercise they skipped, or if they exercised long enough or intensely enough. The list goes on and on. It's impossible to make progress if you're shooting in the dark like that.

What I do with my clients, and what I'll do with you here, is take you through the Stage of Art. We'll cover all of the variables. And once you have a roadmap, it's your job to get and stay on the road. The irony is that the more precise I am with all the variables—timing of meals, portion sizes, ratios of macronutrients, and the duration, intensity, and frequency of exercise—the less time you spend worrying about it. And the faster we see results. It becomes just as routine as brushing your teeth. You probably don't think too much about brushing your teeth. You know you do it without question every night before you go to bed. The same will happen with your eating schedule. You'll know that you have to eat every three to four hours. In fact, your body will start to tell you. And as you become familiar with your plan, you'll know just how much of what you need at every meal.

The beauty of the routine is that you are less likely to be derailed by crises big and small. Because life is a series of crises, big and small. If we wait for everything to be perfect before changing behavior we'll never get anywhere. But if something is a routine, automatic, like a reflex, then we are more likely to see the cumulative effects of those changed behaviors. In fact, when a wrench is thrown into your daily life, there is a certain amount of comfort to be found in maintaining some routines. Just as the samurai knows his technique so well that he simply acts without thought under the threat of imminent death, so, too, should you know your eating and fitness strategy well enough that external pressures should not take you off the track. There should not even be a question of whether or not you're going to exercise five times a week. It is a *given*.

So in the second part of this book, I'll introduce you to people who have reached this Stage of Artlessness. They came to me with Beginner's Mind and were ready to follow their plans from Day One. I'll take you through their progression step by step. You'll see how they learned to take the tools presented in chapters 1 through 16 and elevate their implementation to the cumulative effect of a lifestyle change, one so ingrained that they no longer have to think about it.

Knowing Is Not Enough: The Power of Experience

Reading this book and knowing the material in it is not enough. It is a fundamental principle that Zen cannot be understood without a tangible physical experience. A real-world endeavor through which to learn Zen is required.

As Archbishop Omori Sogen Rotaishi wrote, "Zen without the accompanying physical experience is nothing but empty discussion."[4] So, too, is nutrition information without application. Some of my clients actually think it's enough to show up at my office weekly without doing the homework—without following the food plan and doing the exercise! That's like expecting to become a martial arts expert without practicing. As D. T. Suzuki translated from *Bokkok Kokushi*, "Training in detailed technique is not to be neglected. The understanding of principle alone cannot lead one to the mastery of movements of the body and its limbs."[5] Unfortunately, in today's world of instant gratification, many think it is perfectly reasonable to expect rewards from a half-assed effort. But if that were really possible, why aren't more people satisfied with their fitness status?

For clients, I wish I could somehow impart to them the actual sensation of the physical benefits of *doing* the work. If there were only some way for me to bottle the energy that comes with blood sugar control, the positive shifts in mood that come with an endorphin rush, the knowledge that you can stay with your opponent round for round, the feeling of being light on your feet, or the confidence that comes with being comfortable in your own skin—if only I could capture that feeling and enable non-believers to *feel* it for a second, I think it would be enough to convince them to stay the course.

Unfortunately, that's not quite how it works. Those who are open to a new approach and are willing to take that leap of faith eventually start to feel the benefits of their changed behavior. You'll read the firsthand accounts of those who've experienced incredible change. In the meantime, you will have to take my word and theirs for it until you have experienced the pleasures of a sound mind (and body) for yourself. No one can experience it for you. Nor can anyone else do the work that will bring it to you.

As you progress, then, I ask that you pay special attention to any subtle shifts you might feel in energy, speed, mood, balance, mental awareness, endurance, and, yes, body composition. Many of my clients tell me their energy levels go through the roof only after the first five to seven days of following the plan. Start listening to your body. Become in tune with it, and you'll start to feel the benefits of staying on track. As Zen practitioners will argue, the body itself *is* an experience.

A Dispassionate Approach

As we all know, one of the biggest obstacles to achieving fitness goals is emotional overeating. Again, we could all benefit here from the Zen approach of the samurai. It may seem an odd pairing—the violence of the samurai coupled with a religion known for its compassion. But the directness, practicality, and indifference to life and death, in addition to historical factors, make for a good fit. As Suzuki noted in *Zen and Japanese Culture*, for the samurai, "emotionalities and physical possessions are the heaviest of encumbrances if he wants to conduct himself most efficiently in his vocation."[6] He goes on to say, "you may 'love' or 'hate' anything, but as long as either of the feelings skulks anywhere in your brain, it will somehow color your behavior, and your sword will be affected to that extent."[7]

For those of you who attach food to emotions, you know this all too well. Your emotions—whether positive or negative—will color your behavior, resulting in your turning to food. It would be wise to take a page from the samurai book and view your eating strategy with emotional indifference. This goes hand in hand with the idea of Beginner's Mind. So leave your emotional baggage at the door.

Another point to consider about this dispassionate approach is that no foods are inherently "good" or "bad." I get this all the time: "Is fruit good?" "Is sugar bad?" "Is salt good?" "Is salt bad?" I say, it depends. If you're suffering from hypertension, a high salt intake might not be so great. But if you're in danger of hyponatremia, salt might just save your life! What we say of drugs goes for food as well—"There are no good or bad foods. It's the dose that kills ya."

Be In the Now

Zen teaches us to always be *present* in the moment. You can see how this would have great appeal to the samurai. The presentation of a life or death situation tends to heighten one's awareness. The key to such situations, then, is to concentrate on the work at hand. It makes little sense to worry about the future if you're about to be sliced in half. And so as one of Suzuki's translations states:

> The idea most vital and essential to the samurai is that of death, which he ought to have before his mind day and night, night and day, from dawn of the first day of the year till the last minute of the last day of it. When this notion takes firm hold of you, you are able to discharge your duties to their fullest extent: you are loyal to your master, filial to your parents, and naturally can avoid all kinds of disasters. Not only is your life itself thereby prolonged, but your personal dignity is enhanced.
> Think what a frail thing life is, especially that of a samurai. This being so, you will come to consider every day of your life your last and dedicate it to the fulfillment of your obligations. Never let the thought of a long life seize upon you, for then you are apt to indulge in all kinds of dissipation, and end your days in dire disgrace. This was the reason why Masashige is said to have told his son Masatsura to keep the idea of death all the time before his mind.[8]

Some of you might misinterpret this as an excuse to *carpe diem* it—"Hey, I'm living in the moment. I'm having that milkshake and fries." That's not what I'm saying. In quantum physics, we say the past and future are conceptual illusions. All you have is the moment and in that moment you can decide in what direction you want your life to take. While the future may be an illusion, you can increase the potential of favorable outcomes in the present and *only* in the present.

You should have death in the back of your mind, because in every moment of every day, your body is changing. Contrary to what might be externally perceptible to the human eye, your body is *never* in a static state. You are constantly regenerating red blood cells, which have a lifespan of only 120 days. Our muscles are in a perpetual state of tearing down and reconstruction. You are either doing something harmful or helpful to yourself with every action you take, every minute of every day. Consume too many simple sugars at any given moment, and you cause an immediate insulin surge that leads to the storage of those excess carbs as body fat. Couple just the right amount of carbs with protein, and you're doing something good for yourself by keeping your blood sugar levels humming at an optimal level.

Our body is equipped with an amazing set of signals and mechanisms that keeps it running optimally, but we've become so sensorily overloaded, so distracted, so distanced from our own bodies, that we usually override these signals. We shove food down our throats while we're driving, watching television, or on the phone. Food should be a fundamental joy in life—an experience. Yet, we're usually too distracted to pay attention, both to its consumption and its after–effects. If we really paid attention to how those simple sugars give us a sugar high and crash in the afternoon, we might be less inclined to repeat the process.

In some cases, my clients merely lack the information to get their engines humming. They only need a roadmap. But sometimes it takes a little more attention than that. It's no wonder that Zen monks practice meditation. Studies have shown that Zen monks in meditation exhibited physiological signs of increased awareness— decrease in respiration but increases in pulse and drastic changes in brain wave formation.[9] Rather than being in the pseudo-sleep state that Westerners associate with meditation, advanced meditation brings about an astonishing state of alertness.

I'm not necessarily asking you to meditate daily before and after meals, but start listening to your body. Look for the immediate effects of certain foods on it. Think about its constant state of flux and how your actions and choices are affecting your body *right now*.

Life and Death in Every Bite: "It's a Jungle Out There."

"When you are a martial artist, you only eat what you require and don't get carried away with foods that don't benefit you as a martial artist."[10]

—Bruce Lee

If a samurai went into a swordfight sluggish on cheeseburgers and fries, you might think, "This guy's suicidal." Why would anyone want to run on anything less than the most efficient, clean-burning fuel available? Compared to other sports, the martial arts, of course, are more directly related to the possibility of dire consequences due to poor performance. But in all sports, death—or at least injury —is a risk that can be minimized by maintaining alertness and optimal performance. And diet is necessary to that sharpness.

When your life depends on it, you should have more than enough motivation to do whatever you can to keep the engine humming. The problem is that people often don't make the same connection in their everyday lives. If they're not in immediate danger, they don't necessarily realize that everyday choices are also a matter of life and death. I don't have to tell you that conditions like hypertension, heart disease, certain cancers, diabetes, osteoporosis, and osteoarthritis are attributable to diet.

It's interesting that we don't make this connection between our health and safety in our everyday lives. One of my clients, who works in the inner city, said, "Doing this plan is so important, because it is a *jungle* out there. If you're going around unhealthy, tired, and unaware, you're going to end up in some major trouble." Even I had not attached this kind of urgency to eating well outside the ring, but she's right. If you're wandering around in a stupor because your blood sugars are low or you're in a weakened state because you have nutritional deficiencies, you aren't going to be that sharp, and you may very well be placing yourself at unnecessary risk. Just getting behind the wheel of your car puts you in a potentially hazardous situation.

So if you find yourself on the verge of self-destructive behavior, remember that even though it may not seem like it at the moment, you are always choosing between life and death—or at the very least, between an impaired lifestyle and your best lifestyle. And, of course, if you're a fighter or weapons expert, you've got to be sharp to ensure your safety.

The Art of Expressing the Human Body

"It may be said that Zen uncovers the form of one's True self in the experience of oneness in this physical body."[11]   —Omori Sogen

In Zen Buddhism, there is no disassociation, as there is in the West, between the mind and the external, physical world. How you interact with that physical world is an expression of your being, whatever the endeavor may be—tea ceremony, calligraphy, swordsmanship, and, yes, how you fuel your body. As Kenji Tokitsu explained it, "The reference model for daily gestures that is still taught today in Japan, both in school and at home, has implicit in it that a person will be appreciated for the sincerity with which he puts himself into his gestures entirely. This presupposes that an act can be the total expression of a human being, and that it will be well done if it is done wholeheartedly and implies a relationship with others."[12]

I've discussed at length in other books and magazine articles how crucial this mindset is to the martial arts as well as all physical activity. Bruce Lee referred to it as "the art of expressing the human body." In your tennis serve, basketball shot, golf swing, hook punch, or your dance moves, you are offering a physical representation of yourself.

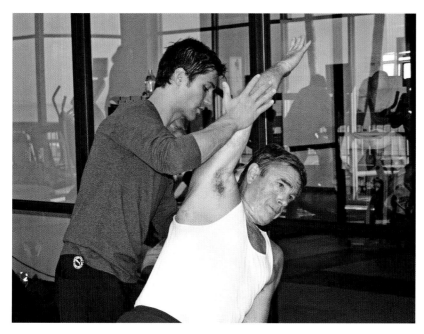

Don't forget, movement itself is a form of expression.

What people may not realize is that they also express themselves in the way they fuel themselves, in the way they treat their own bodies. I occasionally have clients who neglect to take care of their own bodies or sometimes downright abuse them—through undereating, overeating, undertraining, or overtraining. At the root of such problems are usually feelings of inferiority: they may think they are undeserving or unworthy of getting what they want and self-sabotage their programs. Or they may think they are not worth the time and effort required to take care of themselves.

Once you realize that this is not the case—that your well-being *is* a priority—then, of course, your actions must reflect this. Part of that expression is in the way you fuel your body. So every bite, every drink becomes an act of self-respect. You cannot think of eating as deprivation, reward, or a diet.

You need to ask yourself if you are fueling your body in a way that reflects self-respect and acceptance.

Be Like Water

My instructor, Ted Wong, tells a great story of a little homework assignment Bruce Lee once gave him. He asked Ted what is a fighter's most important skill?

> "Speed?" Ted offered.
> "No," was the reply.
> "Technical proficiency?"
> "No."
> "Power!"
> "No. Adaptability."

In his now-famous Pierre Burton interview, Bruce emphasized the importance of adaptability with his water analogy, "I said, 'empty your mind, be formless, shapeless, like water. Now you put water into a cup, it becomes the cup. You put water into a bottle, it becomes the bottle. You put it in a teapot, it becomes the teapot. Now water can flow, or it can crash. Be water, my friend.'" This kind of adaptability is important to a fighter's survival because in the heat of battle, he doesn't have time to think. Nor does he have time (and in most cases, the strength) to force premeditated techniques or strategies on his opponent.

This is a central theme of Zen—that your mind must change with the environment. You must deal with whatever your opponent throws at you. The same can be said of your approach to fueling your body properly. Some of my clients have failed with past plans because of an all-or-nothing mindset. They tried to follow their plan so rigidly that it ended up being impossible to do. If they were a little off for one meal of the day, they'd figure the whole day was shot, and they'd give themselves license to completely fall of the wagon. Every day would end up like this; good start, one mistake, binge.

When clients come to me using this approach, I tell them to look at the big picture: if you make a mistake, just hop back on the wagon and pick up where you left off. We can talk about whatever caused them to derail and I can offer strategies to help them cope the next time.

My client Randy is a great example of someone who adapts to any situation so he can get the job done. As an owner of television stations, Randy is one of my all-time busiest clients. He travels every week, sometimes flying to three or four different cities per week! If he flies into a city at midnight, he's in the hotel gym at 12:30 AM. If he's late for his connecting flight, he's munching on a protein bar as he's running through the airport. I tell my clients who have endless excuses for why they can't meet their fitness goals, "If Randy can do it, the rest of us have no excuses."

If you are truly committed to your fitness, you'll find a way. No gym in the hotel? Get outside and run. Bad weather? Shadowbox for a half hour. Only junk food at a party? Bring some protein powder in a sandwich bag. What this book will do is give you the tools you need to follow your plan anywhere. It should be *easy*. This plan should not be punishing or impossible to do. It is designed to work with your physiology. All of my clients eat out on the road *all* the time. In fact, very few of us cook, including yours truly. But with the information we're presenting here, you should have enough tools in your tool bag to stay on the plan at any restaurant—even the drive-through window.

Lose a Battle, Win the War

I can't tell you how many times I've told my clients my plans are *not* diets. If you want to rebuild your body or to maintain your hard-won results, you need to look at this as a lifestyle and not a quick fix.

Some people only think of their goals in temporary terms. They get to where they want to be for a certain event—competition, wedding, reunion, graduation—and then boomerang to a place that is *worse* than when they started a diet. With that kind of quick fix thinking and transient presence, they are doomed to a life of yo-yo dieting. To me, that just seems like an awful lot of work—not to mention that it's pretty hard on your body.

The samurai cautioned against the one-time victory. So you win one battle. If you don't stay on your game, you might be road kill the next time around. As my dad used to say, "You're only as good as your last win." You can't be smug and rest on your laurels. You must be vigilant and consistent to maintain results.

On the other hand, another self-defeating mentality is the idea that your efforts must be all or nothing. I've had clients who attack their fitness regimes full throttle until they hit one bump in the road. Maybe they have one bad day, or just one bad meal. If they don't achieve perfection, they figure the rest of the program's shot and binge for the next week. So it's one step forward, ten steps back. I tell them they need to readjust their thinking. Again, think big picture. You're in this for the long haul. Like your stock market chart, you're looking for an overall trend. The world doesn't end with one bad day. Of course, if you have two or three bad weeks in a row, we've got a problem. And, yes, in the real world, you have birthdays, holidays, and lost weekends in Vegas. Just get back on that horse and come back better than you were before. You might lose a battle or two, but you'll win the war.

Self-Reliance

It is one of the greatest follies of human nature that we are always looking to outside sources for the answers. We jump from diet to diet, trainer to trainer, book to book, video to video, restaurant to restaurant, hoping that with each novelty, the answer will be thrown into our laps. This is the same for the martial arts, shopping, get-rich-quick schemes, whatever.

The truth is that in almost any endeavor, there are a few basics that you will need to learn from someone else, but from there, you just need to hunker down and do the work. Bruce Lee once wrote that we need to stop looking for secret techniques, that the answer lies in your own body. The same goes for fitness. There are no magic pills. With a few principles and careful control of certain variables, you'll have all the information you need to achieve your goals. Beyond the Stage of Art, the key lies in consistent execution.

This is why I never call my plans "diets." What I devise for my clients is not temporary. Once they've hit their goals, and we've put them on a maintenance plan, they should be able to follow the same plan and principles for the rest of their lives, long after they've walked out of my office for the last time. Similarly, my goal with this book is to give you all the tools necessary to achieve your goals. It's up to you to do the work.

And on that note, I leave you with a passage from Suzuki on self-reliance:

> But in things concerning one's personal experience, all that the master can do is to make the disciples realize that they are now at last in the dark or in the labyrinth and that they must resort to something very much deeper than mere intellection—something which they cannot obtain from another…Intellectual or logical pointer can never be more than a pointer or an onlooker. Personal experience and *Prajna-intuition* are the same thing.[13]

CHAPTER 3

Nutrition Basics

Now that we've addressed some of the motivations for starting and sticking to a fitness lifestyle, the next few chapters will provide the *whys* behind the plans in this book. By knowing the science behind what you'll be doing, you're more likely to adhere to the guidelines in forthcoming chapters.

The Energy Systems

Whether it's running, skipping rope, pumping iron, or drawing a sword, to do any kind of work, your body requires energy. Your cells obtain this energy by incorporating oxygen and the carbon, hydrogen, and oxygen derived from the energy-producing nutrients—carbohydrate, fat, and protein. A high-energy molecule called adenosine triphosphate (ATP) fuels all cells, including your muscle cells. Think of ATP as a form of currency. If I visit Italy from the United States, I can't pay for my prosciutto with U.S. cash. I first have to convert those dollars to euros. Similarly, carbohydrates, fat, and protein do not immediately provide accessible energy once you ingest them. First, just as with those U.S. dollars, they have to be converted to the appropriate currency: they must be broken down and then converted to ATP, a form of energy that the cells can use.

ATP is produced via three systems:

1. The phospho-creatine system
2. The glycolytic system
3. The oxidative system

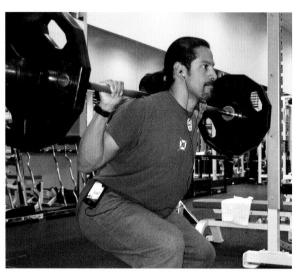

Resistance training employs both the phospho-creatine and glycolytic energy systems.

The Phospho-Creatine System

This is the metabolic system that supplies immediate energy. At any given time, the cells have only a limited supply of ATP stored. To delay the depletion of stored ATP, another molecule called *phospho-creatine* helps rebuild used ATP molecules that have been split. This system does not require oxygen, and is, therefore, an anaerobic process. It can only supply ATP to support all-out effort for 3 to 15 seconds. This would fuel activities like sprinting, weight-training, a shot on goal, a takedown, a kicking combination or a flurry of power punches.

The Glycolytic System (Glycolysis)

For activity exceeding 3 to 15 seconds, cells must switch to the *glycolytic system* to restore the ATP and phospho-creatine supplies that have been depleted. This system provides glucose, a type of sugar that is the major source of fuel to your muscles. The storage form of glucose is called *glycogen*. Two-thirds of your glycogen stores are located in your muscles, and the remaining $1/3$ is stored in your liver. During *glycolysis* glycogen is converted into glucose, which in turn is converted to ATP for energy. This can sustain energy for 2 to 3 minutes. At this point, a high-intensity all-out effort will exceed the body's ability to supply enough oxygen to produce ATP. When insufficient oxygen is available, lactic acid is produced. You know that burning in your delts by the end of a 3-minute round? That's the unpleasant sensation of lactic acid buildup. Keep it up and the lactic acid and glycogen depletion will eventually prevent you from throwing out any more jabs.

Wrestling is largely anaerobic, requiring short bursts of explosive energy for controls and escapes. To restore the phospho-creatine and glycogen stores, a 3- to 5-minute rest period is required. But fighters only get *one* minute of rest between rounds! Yes, and that's why we have the oxidative system.

The Oxidative System

The *oxidative system* allows for a much greater production of ATP than the anaerobic (phospho-creatine and glycolytic) systems. Through conditioning and sound dietary practices, you can increase the efficiency with which your cells use oxygen to produce ATP. This will delay the onset of lactic buildup, and, consequently, the onset of muscle fatigue. Sports like boxing and mixed martial arts require multiple rounds of continuous movement but provide insufficient rest to restore systems of anaerobic metabolism. Therefore, the oxidative system, or aerobic metabolism, will enable you to go the distance. Oxygen is a necessary ingredient in the chemical pathway that churns out large numbers of ATP molecules.

The Three Systems in Multiple-Sprint Sports

It is important to note that all three systems are used in the martial arts. The phospho-creatine and glycolytic systems provide immediate energy for high-intensity work. For example, they may help you get through the first round. This gives the oxidative system time to get up and running. Once this occurs, all three processes may overlap each other. Basic footwork, moving around the ring, and maintaining position in relation to your opponent are mostly supported by aerobic metabolism. But shooting out a stiff jab, launching a combination, and quickly evading an attack require fast, explosive energy. That's where the phospho-creatine and glycolytic systems come in. They may be called upon in the midst of aerobic activity.

The martial arts, like other multiple-sprint sports, now require training to improve the capabilities of each of the three systems. Balancing these training modes and the nutrients to support them will be addressed later on. Just keep in mind that strength and power training will involve the phospho-creatine and glycolytic systems. Cardiovascular training such as running, skipping rope, shadowboxing, and multiple rounds in the ring will develop endurance and your ability to utilize the aerobic system.

The Six Nutrients: An Overview

Nutrients are substances that must be ingested and are required for our bodies to run efficiently and effectively. There are six categories of nutrients. They are vitamins, minerals, carbohydrates, protein, fat, and water. While all six play roles in energy-producing chemical pathways, only three are actual sources of *energy*. We call these three the *macronutrients*, and they are carbohydrates, protein, and fat. The macronutrients provide the actual hydrogen, carbon, and oxygen atoms that go through the metabolic pathways to produce ATP, our energy currency. When supplement dealers tell you their vitamin and mineral products will give you extra energy, know that this is not technically the case. Only the macronutrients are actual sources of energy.

This doesn't mean, however, that the micronutrients are not important to energy production. Vitamins and minerals may not be fuel sources, but they make metabolic reactions possible. Still, if you don't consume enough sources of energy in proper ratios, those vitamins and minerals will have nothing to do—they won't have any macronutrients to work on.

The sixth nutrient is water. Our bodies are two-thirds water, so it's no surprise that this is the medium through which oxygen, nutrients, and waste products are transported.

The Macronutrients: High Carb vs. High Protein

In recent years a battle has been raging between those who advocate high-carbohydrate diets and those who promote high-protein diets. Actually, the battle lines were first drawn in the 1960s when Dr. Atkins introduced his high animal protein and animal fat diet. Since then, however, the majority of professional health organizations have fallen on the side of high-carbohydrate diets. The American Dietetic Association, American Diabetes Association, American Heart Association, and United States Department of Agriculture, which constructed the Food Guide Pyramid, all originally recommend a diet that consists of 45% to 65% carbohydrate.

Despite these endorsements of high-carb diets, the 1990s were marked by a resurgence of low-carb/high protein diets, demonstrated by the book sales of *Enter the Zone, Dr. Atkins' New Diet Revolution, Sugar Busters,* and a plethora of similar books touting the evils of carbohydrates. They recommend a diet that derives 40% or less of its calories from carbohydrates. While many of these books base this recommendation on erroneous "science," new studies spurred by the controversy have found evidence that such diets may help with weight loss.

So who's right? Well, as in any area of medicine or the health industry, when it comes to nutrition, we always run into the variable of human individuality. We come in all different shapes and sizes, and sometimes those shapes and sizes are a result of the different ways in which our bodies process the food we eat. I've had clients who lose body fat very easily. Others lose very slowly. Some are hard gainers. Others would give away their muscle if they could. Everyone seems to have different areas where they either gain muscle or store fat more easily than others. Some fighters I've worked with do well with very little carbohydrate. Others need more to perform optimally. So even though we might be under the impression that dietary guidelines are cut and dried, like most things in life, it's just not that simple.

Keep in mind, then, that the guidelines in this book are a mere starting point, from which you will later customize your plan. I am giving you the tools to monitor your progress and make the necessary changes based on your progress.

As with everything in life, balance is key. Without enough macronutrients, vitamins and minerals are rendered worthless. Inadequate vitamins and minerals, in turn, will result in inefficient energy production. Excessive vitamin and mineral intake, however, may be dangerous. Any of the macronutrients taken in excess will be stored as fat. Insufficient fluids will hinder energy production and waste removal. Too much can lead to dangerously low levels of electrolytes. You get the idea. Now let's look at each of the nutrient categories in a little more detail.

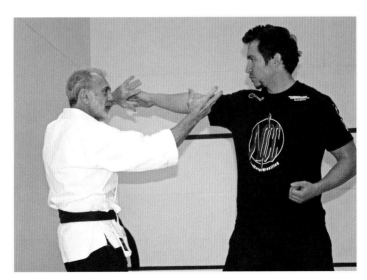

Carbohydrates are necessary for staying mentally sharp during extended bouts of exercise.

CHAPTER 4

Carbohydrates

Safety in Carbs

Sports nutrition has, for the most part, focused on endurance sports like distance running, swimming, and cycling. There is usually quite a bit of time for endurance athletes to recover between such events. Much attention is also given to the pre-event diet, while strategies for recovery are often ignored. Martial artists, however, are not solely endurance athletes. Boxing and mixed martial arts, for example, combine explosive anaerobic activity (e.g., for takedowns and throwing combinations at near-maximal exertion) and aerobic endurance (to last multiple rounds). Martial arts also can be practiced year round. There is no off-season for recovery.

Supplemental training may require daily weight and aerobic workouts in addition to skills development. All this training can result in symptoms of sluggishness (both mental and physical), weakness, loss of concentration, and loss of coordination. Sports nutritionists collectively refer to these symptoms as "staleness." To understand staleness, you must first understand that the main source of fuel to your muscles, and the *only* source of fuel to your brain, is glucose. All carbohydrates are eventually converted to glucose, which may be available for immediate use by your brain and muscles. They may also be stored as glycogen in the muscles and liver. When needed, glycogen is then converted back to glucose.

As we just mentioned, glucose is the only source of fuel to your brain, which means that your diet not only affects how well you function in your daily life, but your judgment and reaction in the ring as well. Research has shown that athletes' motor skills are impaired when their carbohydrate intake is low. Not something you want to happen when you need to be weaving and bobbing out of harm's way. Trainers often drag their clients into my office when clients have near-fainting spells during training. Usually the culprit is low blood sugar. Obviously, it's not a good idea to be lacking in carbohydrates, but for martial artists, it's downright dangerous. It's hard enough having an opponent who is trying to knock you out. Don't help him!

Sources

Put simply, carbohydrates are foods that have plant origins. This would include fruits, vegetables, legumes, and grains. An easy way to remember this is to know that if it comes from a plant, it's a source of carbohydrates. If it comes from an animal, it does *not* provide carbohydrates. For example, you don't get carbohydrates from an egg. Comes from a chicken, right? Nor would you get carbs from a steak. The one exception would be milk and yogurt, which do contain significant amounts of carbohydrates in addition to protein.

Sports drinks, shakes and sports bars are certainly acceptable sources of carbohydrates, but because there is such a wide range of products, you need to watch out for the ratios of protein, carb, and fat. Also keep in mind that, unless fortified, they do not provide the additional nutrients that whole foods do—like the vitamins, minerals, and fiber you would get from fruit, or the calcium you would get from dairy products. If you are going to use sports products, do not use them as your main source of carbohydrates. Choose whole grains, fresh fruits and vegetables. Otherwise, you'll miss out on other good things like vitamins, minerals, fiber, antioxidants, and phytochemicals, all of which bolster your general health and play a role in protection against heart disease and cancer.

Types of Carbohydrates

You may have also heard of complex and simple carbohydrates. Simple carbohydrates are made of either single or double molecules. These are called monosaccharides and disaccharides, respectively. Glucose is a monosaccharide.

Complex carbohydrates, on the other hand, are long chains of sugar molecules. In plants, sugars are stored as starch, which is a complex carbohydrate. Fiber is also a complex carbohydrate, but it is not digestible by the human body.

The Glycemic Index: A Useful Tool?

The glycemic index is a scale that indicates how quickly an individual food is broken down, converted to glucose, and then moved into the blood. Glucose, which does not require any conversion, is assigned the highest rating. Foods assigned higher numbers are converted to glucose and raise blood sugar levels faster than foods with lower glycemic index ratings.

Armed with this terminology, you may think that simple carbohydrates may automatically have a higher glycemic index (GI). Many diet books will tell you complex carbs are better because they provide more lasting energy, since they take longer to convert to glucose. Makes sense, but this isn't always the case. For instance, apple juice has a GI of 45, while watermelon has a GI of 103. Both are simple carbohydrates! Or consider potatoes with a GI of 116 and green peas with a GI of 50. Both of these are complex carbohydrates. To futher complicate matters, consider that just ½ cup of apple juice delivers 15 grams of carbohydrate. But a full 1½ cup of watermelon delivers the same 15 grams of carb. To account for both glycemic index and portion size, Harvard University developed a new scale called the glycemic load. For a comprehensive database of both glycemic index and glycemic load, visit www.glycemicindex.com.

What makes the glycemic index of limited use, though, is the fact that it's a scale for *individual* foods. There are many other factors that contribute to the time it takes glucose to hit your blood. The presence of fat, protein, and soluble fiber may slow this process. Since most of us eat foods in combination with other foods, this combination is a more influential factor on blood glucose than the glycemic index. Low cooking temperature, ripeness, or processing may also increase the time it takes for carbohydrates to spike your blood sugars.

In a later chapter, we'll discuss how the ratios of carb to protein to fat, and not the glycemic index, are the real keys to blood sugar control.

Carbohydrates for Recovery and Preparation

As mentioned above, carbohydrates are either converted to glucose and immediately used or are converted to a storage form called glycogen. Some of it is stored in the liver, but most of it is stored in skeletal muscle.

The catch is that we can only store limited amounts of carbohydrate as glycogen. While the amount of storage is partially influenced by your level of conditioning, the maximum is only about 500–600 grams of carbohydrate at any given time.

If you exercise an hour or less a day, you probably do not have to take special care to replenish your glycogen stores. However, if you exercise longer than this, you may be depleting them. When significantly depleted, you will no longer be able to exercise. This is popularly referred to as "hitting the wall."

Remember if you exercise for over an hour on successive days or several times in a single day, you will dip further and further into your glycogen reserves. Not allowing your body to catch up by either resting or monitoring your diet will result in cumulative glycogen depletion. You will poop out sooner because less fuel is available to your muscles and—voila! You have staleness and wall hitting.

The key to avoiding staleness, then, is to replenish your glycogen stores with carbohydrates. To maximize glycogen storage, the following must be taken into account: timing of carbohydrate ingestion, rate of digestion, and, of course, amount of carbohydrate. In general, you want to get carbohydrates—as well as some protein—into your system following a workout. There is a window in which your body is most efficient at replenishing its glycogen stores. During the first 15 minutes after exercise, your levels of hormones that mobilize glycogen into glucose conversion—epinephrine, norepinephrine, and cortisol—diminish. After that, your body releases a different hormone, glycogen synthase, to help you replenish glycogen stores quickly. It makes your body a glucose sponge so that any carbohydrates are readily absorbed and stored as glycogen. The window of time when glycogen synthase levels are highest is between 15 minutes and 2 hours after your workout.

The type of carbohydrates you ingest at this time is also important. For recovery, you will want to ingest carbohydrates that are rapidly absorbed by your bloodstream. Many factors can affect the rate of carbohydrate absorption, including texture, degree of processing, presence of fiber, starch content, and interaction with protein and fat. In general, slowly absorbed carbohydrates are good choices prior to exercise, while rapidly and moderately absorbed ones are better for glycogen replenishment. So before a workout, you may consider either a low-glycemic-index food item, or you may want to combine a higher-glycemic-index item with a serving of protein to slow absorption. In this way, you put together a low-glycemic-index *meal*. A post-workout meal that includes some protein has been shown to result in faster muscle recovery as well.

Also remember that after exercise, many athletes may not feel like eating immediately following rigorous activity. If this is the case, a liquid source of carbohydrate, like Gatorade, is a good choice. This is also a good time to use other sports supplements like gels and sports bars, which are more easily tolerated after exercise.

How Much Carbohydrate Do I Need?

Determining carbohydrate requirements is tricky business. The often-recommended intake for athletes is 7 to 10 grams of carbohydrate per kilogram of body weight. In my experience with clients, I find this is too much. For body fat loss and maintenance, I've had very good results with my clients in the 75 to 200 g/day range, but this will vary depending on a wide number of factors.

Once again, everyone is different. Your goals, amount of activity, type of activity, body type, and hereditary factors will all influence the amount of carbohydrate you need. I prefer to find out the total number of calories required and then make sure protein needs are taken care of first. Carbohydrate and fat requirements are factored in afterward.

Carbohydrate needs can be highly variable so what I prefer to do, instead of giving a cut-and-dried formula, is to first determine total energy requirements. From there, I'd use one of the daily calorie templates in this book and then monitor your body composition.

If you're gaining fat and muscle, we'll scale back your calories, and carbs will be the first thing to go. If you're losing both muscle and fat, I would increase your protein. If you're losing muscle and gaining fat, I would increase your overall calories by 250–500 and this would include the addition of carbohydrates. And, of course, in most cases, if you're losing fat and gaining muscle, then we wouldn't have to make any changes—that's exactly what we want!

The important thing to remember is to first calculate your total caloric and protein needs. Then, based on your body composition, you can adjust the carbohydrates, but in general, they are the most expendable of the macronutrients.

A Note for All You Muscle Builders

While it's true that I like to center my plans around protein, as with all aspects of nutrient intake, more is *not* always better. Yes, your body needs a certain amount of protein, and we'll discuss that in Chapter 5. And, yes, athletes tend to need more than the general population does. But it is not protein itself that causes the building of new muscle. Strength training, which means increasing the workload that muscles must perform, is what causes muscle growth. And what is the fuel that enables muscles to do this work? Carbohydrates. Remember carbohydrates are the main source of fuel for your muscles, and they are the only clean-burning fuel for muscles. Protein merely provides the building blocks, or structural materials.

If the carbohydrate supply is insufficient, through a series of metabolic pathways, your body can convert some protein to glucose, and then energy. This process is called *gluconeogenesis*, and it comes at the expense of maintaining and/or building your lean body tissue—in other words, your muscles. With insufficient energy intake, your body will literally eat itself by feeding on your muscle tissue. And with insufficient carbohydrate intake, your body will use for energy, protein that would be put to better use for muscle building and repair. In this way, carbohydrates have a muscle-sparing effect. They provide fuel so your body can use protein for building and maintaining muscle mass.

"Fat Burns in a Flame of Carbohydrate"

The actual metabolic pathway that this phrase describes is too detailed for the scope of this book (remember the Krebs cycle from high school biology?), but simply put, it means that carbohydrate is the cleanest-burning fuel for our bodies. Remember from our nutrition basics in Chapter 3 that the aerobic system yields the most ATP or energy. When this system kicks in, we dip into our fat stores for energy. But in order for this to occur, some carbohydrate must also be available, because there is a molecule derived from carbohydrates that makes fat burning possible.

True, through gluconeogenesis, you may convert protein to glucose, but this results in a condition called ketosis. An inadequate carbohydrate supply results in only partial fat breakdown and an accumulation of byproducts called ketones. This is why we say carbohydrates provide clean-burning fuel. Carbohydrate availability prevents the buildup of potentially harmful byproducts like ketones. Not only is ketosis detrimental to athletic performance, but it may also threaten your general health, resulting in dehydration, electrolyte imbalance, exacerbation of existing kidney conditions, loss of lean tissue, and blood lipid elevation.

Don't Leave Your Fight (or Your Carbs) on the Road

You hear this phrase describing over-trained boxers all the time. Besides the obvious structural wear and tear that occurs with overtraining, excessive physical activity can deplete your glycogen stores, leaving you stale and with no fuel to your muscles. Take this one step further, and your body will dip into your protein stores (your lean muscle tissue) to provide energy. In a French study, judoists on low carb diets exhibited increased levels of extracellular markers of muscle catabolism (that

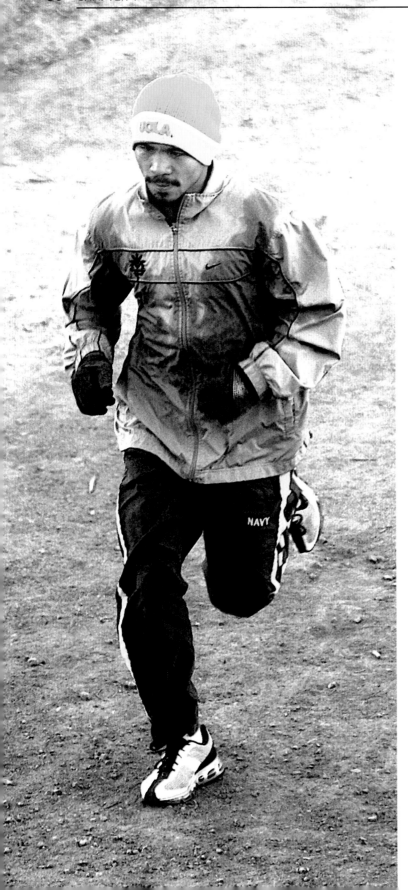

is, muscle destruction) following a match.[14] Not good for fighters who need that muscle mass for speed and power. This principle also supports the general training strategy of not running more than a few miles at a time. Long distance runners, in contrast, experience an adaptation whereby their bodies resist keeping and adding muscle tissue. So unless you're planning on running from your opponent, it's a good idea to get enough carbohydrates.

Carbs During Exercise

Now that you know all about staleness, wall hitting, and the protein-sparing effect of carbohydrates, you can probably guess the advantages of ingesting carbohydrates during physical activity. Chances are that you're exercising more than one hour a day and/or exercising on successive days. In addition to practicing the specifics of their particular art, most martial artists include resistance training and cardiovascular programs in their training. If this

Manny Pacquiao's training includes running, as well as careful balance of nutrient intake. Carbohydrate intake during extended bouts of exercise has been proven to improve performance. *(Photo: Kazumichi)*

is the case, you're going to want to keep those glycogen stores as elevated as possible. We've already talked about how to do this when recovering from exercise, but there are also steps you can take *during* exercise.

When you ingest carbohydrates during exercise, you provide glucose to your body, so that you'll minimize the extent to which you must dip into your glycogen stores. This will help you maintain your energy, concentration, and performance level for a longer period of time, and will delay the time it takes for you to fatigue. Carbohydrate supplementation is well documented in sports science literature. In study after study, carbohydrate supplementation has been shown to delay the onset of fatigue—on treadmills and cycles. Subjects given carbohydrate feedings while cycling were able to continue 33 minutes longer than the placebo group.[15] Many other studies have shown that carbohydrate ingestion during exercise delays time to fatigue significantly. In addition to endurance advantages, carbohydrate ingestion has shown improvement in performance in simulated hockey and tennis studies.

So how much carb are we talking? Studies to date show a range of 30 to 60 grams of carbohydrate per hour of exercise can yield performance and endurance benefits. Solid foods or liquids may supply this carbohydrate. This is a matter of individual preference and tolerance. Some like the satiety that solid foods provide. Others may find solids too difficult to tolerate during exercise and may prefer liquid supplements like Gatorade and Powerade. Liquids empty from the stomach more rapidly and simultaneously replace fluids lost with perspiration. Gels also provide an easily digested source of carbohydrates and they're more portable than liquids.

And while carbohydrate-protein drinks may reduce muscle damage during exercise,[16] they do not enhance endurance capacity. In a study by Van Essen and Gibala, cycling performance time was identical for subjects taking the carbohydrate-only and carbohydrate-protein drinks.[17]

Liquid Supplements

If you do decide to go with a liquid supplement, there are a few things you should know. First, the concentration of the sports drink should be around 4–8%. The American College of Sports Medicine recommends replacing fluids and supplying carbohydrates with 600–1200 mL or 20–40 oz of 4–8% solution every hour. If possible, you may want to distribute this amount by ingesting 5–10 oz every 15 to 20 minutes.

For example, Gatorade has a 6% concentration, which is 14g carbohydrate per 8 oz. Accelerade has 7% concentration at 17g carbohydrate per 8 oz. To avoid gastrointestinal distress, then, you may want to add 8 oz of water to 8 oz of these supplements.

Also note that some studies have shown that a concentration higher than 6.9% may result in gastrointestinal distress. For this reason, if you are using a sports drink to replace fluid losses as well, you may want to dilute it, so that the concentration is not too high. Also, if one of your goals is to lose body fat, you may want to forego or minimize the extra calories you'll receive from a liquid supplement. There is often a tradeoff between performance and weight loss. Weigh your goals and priorities and proceed from there.

Another factor you will want to consider when choosing a sports drink is the source of carbohydrate. Fructose has been shown to cause gastrointestinal distress in studies, so you may want to avoid fruit juices and other drinks high in fructose. This is probably because fructose must first be converted to glycogen in the liver. The extra time required to convert to glucose may result in gastrointestinal discomfort. Gatorade and similar drinks contain glucose and sucrose, which are better bets for improving tolerance.

Carbs Before a Workout

A pre-workout meal of both carbs and protein is a good place to start. In general this is about a 2 to 1 protein-to-carb ratio. This should be ingested 1 to 2 hours before exercise. If you need something closer to your workout, consider a smaller snack in the same proportion 30 minutes prior to exercise. Or you might try a sports drink just before your workout.

Aim to provide a steady supply of carbohydrate throughout your workout. You may want to refer to the glycemic index and choose foods low on the scale. Or, as suggested earlier, create a low glycemic index *meal* with protein. Remember that other factors like fat, fiber, cooking methods, and cooking times will affect how fast that glucose hits your blood.

A Final Word on Carbs

In recent years, carbohydrates have been unfairly demonized as the nutrient responsible for weight gain, mood swings, fatigue, and other ills. True, if there's any nutrient we tend to overdo, it would be carbs, but they are not the enemy. For fighters, they're key to maintaining energy levels, building muscle, concentration, performance, and to a certain extent, fat burning. Do *not* neglect them. As with any sport, carbohydrates will help you prevent injuries by maintaining your performance and concentration. It's no coincidence that most athletic injuries occur in the latter stages of competition when glycogen stores have been depleted. Furthermore, keep in mind that the martial arts have their roots in life or death situations. Their original purpose was to do damage. This potentially makes these sports more dangerous than others. As Jeff Silverman writes, "Boxers fight and fighters box. Nobody plays boxing, like they play ball or golf, because boxing isn't something to play around with"—nor is any combat sport. Because of this, you'll want to keep your mental alertness and physical prowess as elevated as possible, and carbohydrates in the proper amounts make this possible.

Manny Pacquiao sparring. Carbohydrates are key to fueling your alertness and skill, whether you're training or competing. *(Photo: Kazumichi)*

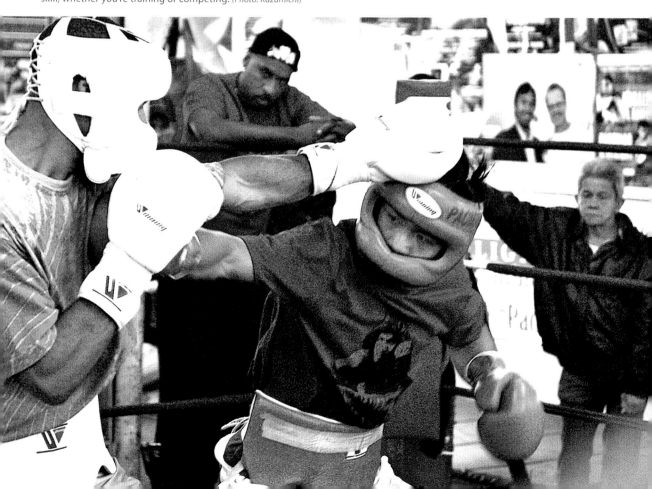

CHAPTER 5

Protein

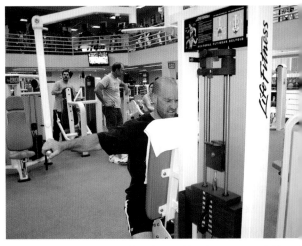

Protein provides the raw material for m[...]
building and mainten[...]

Protein Building Blocks

The importance that athletes place on protein is not so much overemphasized as it is misplaced. Yes, protein is absolutely necessary for our bodies to function. It is needed for proper tissue building and maintenance. This includes building and repair of hair, skin, nails, and of most interest to athletes, muscle. Protein is also required for regulation of some of our most basic systems. Hormones, enzymes, nutrient carriers, and antibodies are all composed of proteins.

The misconception, however, that athletes have regarding protein is that protein itself builds muscle. To be more precise, carbohydrate fuels the building of muscle, while protein provides the raw structural material of muscle. A detailed description of how muscles grow can be found in many bodybuilding and kinesiology books. The basic principle, though, is that our bodies adapt to stresses we place on them. When we lift more weight than we are accustomed to lifting, out muscles are subject to micro injuries and tears. The body responds by rebuilding the injured muscle into a bigger, stronger muscle in anticipation of dealing with greater workloads. We call this growth hypertrophy.

This is the reason why athletes gaining muscle tissue and individuals supporting tissue building (e.g., children, pregnant women, etc.) need more protein. They need more *raw materials*. The additional amount of protein required for growth, however, varies widely depending on the individual. When I have a fighter either trying to gain weight or lose some bulk, protein is one of the primary nutrients we manipulate. We'll get into specifics later in the chapter.

For now, think of it this way: protein provides your lumber, your nuts and bolts—the raw materials. It does not provide an efficient fuel for assembly of those raw materials. And it does not provide the best energy source for fueling your muscles. Eating protein without carbohydrate is like having a bunch of loose boards and screws, but no electricity to power the drill.

Nevertheless, you still need those raw materials for structural building and repair, so let's talk about what exactly protein is and where you can find it in your diet.

Amino Acids

Like our other macronutrients, protein consists of carbon, hydrogen, and oxygen. Structurally speaking, though, what differentiates protein from carbohydrate or fat is that protein also contains about 16% nitrogen. Nitrogen is the key component of the most basic unit of proteins, the amino acid. Different amino acids can be linked in an infinite number of sequences to form different structures. One sequence of amino acids might form the protein for a specific hormone, while another combination of amino acids will provide a structural unit for muscle, and yet another combination might contribute to the formation of an enzyme.

When we eat protein, it is broken down into its constituent amino acids. These are then used to synthesize various proteins that the body needs. Our body can synthesize some amino acids. We call these nonessential amino acids. The 12 non-essential amino acids are alanine, cysteine, glycine, arginine, asparagine, cystine, proline, serine, aspartic acid, glutamic acid, glutamine, and tyrosine.

There is a group of amino acids, however, that we cannot synthesize. These must be obtained from external sources—otherwise known as food! These are called essential amino acids, meaning they are an essential part of our diet. The essential amino acids are isoleucine, leucine, lysine, methionine, phenylalaline, threonine, valine, and tryptophan. For children, histidine is also an essential amino acid.

Protein Sources and Quality

Protein sources that contain a balanced ratio of essential amino acids in amounts adequate to support good health are said to be complete. Animal sources provide complete protein. That means anything that has a face, walks, runs, crawls, swims, or flies provides complete protein. By the way, we're talking about fresh animal sources, *not* processed meats like bologna, sausage, bacon, or salami. These have protein, but they aren't exactly the best sources and also have things that you *don't* want, like fat and nitrites. Processed foods use the terms "all beef" or "all chicken" rather loosely, which can mean the inclusion of lips, teeth, bones, hair, tails, etc., recalling the 1980s ad campaign "parts is parts."

Another measure of protein quality is its biological value (BV). Proteins that are best digested, absorbed, and retained are said to have high biological value. This means that most of the nitrogen is retained and not excreted by the body. Eggs have been assigned a biological value of 100 meaning 100% of egg white protein is retained by the body. Dairy and soy products both provide complete protein. But dairy has high BV, while soy does not. The nitrogen portion goes right through you.

An important point to make here is that just because you want to build muscle, doesn't mean you automatically must take in more protein. Many people already eat much more protein than they need. Second, the body adapts to strength training. Just as your body rebuilds muscle bigger and stronger each time it recovers from those little tears, your body also gets better at retaining the nitrogen needed to build those muscles.

A Note for Vegans

Vegetarianism is a subject worthy of its own book, but we'll briefly address it here. If you are a vegetarian, you can still get the equivalent of a complete protein by combining certain plant foods, but the biological value of that complete array of amino acids does little good because the nitrogen portion gets excreted.

This goes for soy as well. And because soy is comprised of phytoestrogens, if you're a guy, this could result in hormonal imbalances that could throw your testosterone levels out of whack, making it difficult to build and retain muscle tissue. Soy in moderation should be fine, but do not use it as your main protein source, and if you are very lean and trying to get leaner and/or add muscle, I would avoid it altogether.

While vegetarians may be able to take in sufficient amounts of all the amino acids, vegans who eat no animal products (including no dairy and eggs) could be at risk for zinc, vitamin B_{12}, and iron deficiency. This could result in a variety of problems including compromised immune function and anemia. Also, because of the literal pounding that many martial artists take—whether it's taking body shots in the ring or getting whacked regularly with a shinai—I strongly urge you to incorporate some kind of high BV protein into your diet for structural repair as well as immune function.

You do not, of course, have to chomp on animal flesh to get high BV protein. Egg whites, cottage cheese, whey protein powder, and fish, to name a few, are all great alternatives to chicken or beef. If you are not entirely vegan for ethical reasons, then I urge you to go to these alternative sources.

Excess Protein

Let's face it, competitive athletes have many opportunities to overdo things, so it's important to remember that more is not necessarily better. Training may be good for you, but too much training can leave you tired, injured, or burnt out. The same goes for your diet. Food is good for you, but overeating can leave you with a spare tire.

Unlike carbohydrate, which can be stored in limited amounts as glycogen, protein cannot be stored when taken in excess. Once the body has the protein it needs for maintaining health and muscle tissue, the excess must undergo a process called deamination. This means that the nitrogen-containing component of an amino acid must be removed and then excreted by the kidneys. The excess nitrogen must be excreted to maintain your body's acid-base balance, which is essential for your survival.

Keep in mind that any of the three macronutrients taken in excess gets stored as fat. Too much carbohydrate gets stored as fat. Too much protein gets stored as fat. Too much fat gets stored as fat. Even if you increase your protein intake and do not gain body fat, you may end up with more muscle than you want, which can make you bulkier and slower. As with everything in this book, it's a fine edge we're always walking between sufficient intake and excess. Know what you want to achieve and then be sure to monitor your progress.

Let's Talk Numbers

Now that I've told you there is an optimal range for your daily protein intake, it's time to talk specifics. You'll hear it again and again in this book, but here goes. The numbers and ranges presented here serve as a guideline based on years of scientific research, but when we talk nutrition, as with shoes, one size does not fit all. In addition, your protein requirement is based on a number of factors, including body composition goals, training schedule and modes, as well as where you stand today. The numbers here will give you a starting point. For best results, you should have your body fat measured by a registered dietitian who can then make diet modifications based on your progress and changing goals.

Let's get started.

The Daily Recommended Intake (please see the vitamin section for an explanation of the DRIs) for the average person who exercises moderately is 0.8 grams of protein per kilogram of body weight. Research has established, however, that athletes engaged in activity of higher intensity need more protein than this. While some research has claimed that at 2.4 grams of protein per kilogram, muscle growth is no longer aided by further increases in protein, I've had plenty of clients who actually needed more than this to increase their muscle mass. Some have been successful with amounts as high as 3.5 g/kg.

Once again, the answers lie with the individual. To really know how much protein is needed, you'll want to have your body composition monitored weekly. If you're losing muscle and fat, you need to increase protein only. If you're losing muscle and gaining fat, you need to increase your overall calories, including those that come from protein.

When it comes to protein and the martial arts, it's essential that you get enough high BV protein. It has been shown that athletes who participate in high impact, contact sports suffer microtrauma to muscles and connective tissues. Adequate protein is necessary to repair these injuries. Anyone who's pounded the heavy bag, practiced falls on the mat, or taken a licking with a kendo shinai knows there's a lot of wear and tear involved. But also remember that while you need enough protein, drastically exceeding the required amount will hurt you more than it will help you.

Do the Math

Now you have the numbers. Let's try an example. Say we have a 135-pound fighter who needs 2.8 g protein/kg. To convert weight in pounds to weight in kilograms, we divide by 2.2. So,

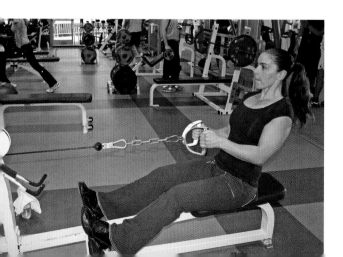

135 pounds ÷ 2.2 = 61 kilograms

61 kilograms x 2.8 grams protein per kilogram body weight = 170.8 grams protein

So our fighter's daily protein requirement would be 170.8 grams of protein.

Your protein requirements are dependent on the specifics of your training program and your body composition test results.

It's your turn. First convert your body weight in pounds to kilograms.

1. _____ ÷ 2.2 = _____ kg
(your body weight in pounds)

2. _____ x 2.8 g protein/kg body weight = _____ g protein
(answer from Step 1)

Now suppose we have a competitive athlete who is taking a break from training specifically for his sport/art but is still engaging in weight and aerobic training. Then we would use a number between 1.6 and 1.8 grams of protein per kilogram body weight. So if our athlete weighs 70 kg, we could give him 1.8 grams of protein per kilogram of body weight:

70 kg body weight x 1.8 g protein/kg body weight = 126 g protein

When he goes back to heavy training for his sport, we would bump his daily protein requirement back up to 2.8 grams per kg.

70 kg body weight x 2.8 g protein/kg body weight = 196 g protein

Got it? Later, we'll show you how 196 grams of protein translates into real-world food portions. We'll also pull all this information together in meal plan templates, which will make getting started a little easier.

Timing

Remember how we recommended a 2:1 ratio of protein to carbs immediately following exercise? You already know why the carbs are important. Well, the protein is, too, because the combination of the two accelerates the uptake of glucose into cells and the synthesis of glycogen. Protein taken with carbohydrate also induces the release of growth hormone, which is pivotal to muscle building. That 2:1 ratio taken within 15 minutes to 2 hours after exercise is crucial to the refueling, maintenance, and growth of your muscles.

CHAPTER 6

Fat

The Nutrient with a Bad Rap

Like carbohydrates, fat has gotten a bad rap. Overconsumption of fat can cause you all kinds of problems, but so can *any* other nutrient taken in excess. Too many carbs get stored as fat. Too much protein gets stored as fat. Too much fat gets stored as fat. All roads lead to fat. The bottom line is that when you consume more calories than you expend the excess goes into storage. More precisely, 3500 excess calories equals one pound of fat.

To be fair, though, let's remind ourselves of all the good things fat does. First, it allows you to absorb certain vitamins that must be dissolved in fat before they can be used by your body. These include vitamins A, D, E, and K. Fats help maintain

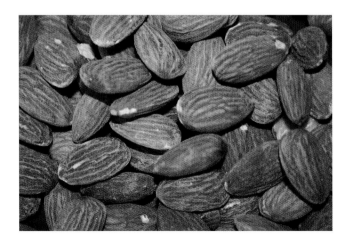

Nuts are a great source
of healthy fat.

blood pressure and triglyceride and cholesterol levels. They maintain skin and cell membrane health. They're involved in regulating immune function. Fat also is a major component of the brain so it's not surprising that the kinds of fats you eat have an influence on your brain's composition and ability to function. And since we can store glycogen and protein in limited quantities, fat, which is a concentrated storage form of energy, is what enables us to spar on the mat for multiple rounds and go the distance in the ring.

Those are the good things fat can do for you, so why has it been our most-maligned nutrient? Well, as we said, just like every nutrient, you can have too much of a good thing. Compared to other energy-providing nutrients, fat is the most nutrient dense. Protein and carbohydrate provide 4 calories per gram. Alcohol provides 7 calories. And fat provides a whopping 9 calories. Fat fulfills a lot of important functions, but when you take in more than you need, you end up keeping it.

Types of Fat

Any discussion of fat is a little like Word Soup, but the truth is that not all fats are created equal. So let's learn a little vocabulary first.

Triglycerides

Triglycerides are fats found in food and in your body. When you eat any of the macronutrients, whether they're protein, carbohydrate, or fat, your liver goes to work and converts them into triglycerides. This is how fat is stored in your body. High triglycerides have been correlated with higher risk for heart disease. To make matters worse, triglycerides signal the liver to produce more cholesterol. Dietary fat always gets a bad rap, but alcohol and concentrated sugars elevate your triglyceride levels as well, so fat's not the only nutrient you've got to watch.

Cholesterol

Next up is cholesterol. There's a lot of misunderstanding about cholesterol. First, dietary cholesterol is only derived from animal products, specifically, animal fat. So if it's fat from something that walks, swims, flies, or crawls, it's going to give you some cholesterol. If not, then it comes from a plant, which is cholesterol free.

Cholesterol that you get from food, by the way, is different from the cholesterol that your body produces, which is called blood or serum cholesterol.

Two types of blood cholesterol are HDL (high-density lipoprotein) and LDL (low-density lipoprotein). HDL cholesterol transports cholesterol away from your blood vessels to the liver for repackaging or excretion. It's like the garbage truck that picks up your trash and takes it away from your house. That's why you may have heard it referred to as the "good" cholesterol. It takes cholesterol *away* from your arteries.

LDL cholesterol, on the other hand, brings cholesterol to various parts of the body. Think of LDL cholesterol as a delivery truck dropping off cholesterol to your cells and arteries. In excessive amounts, it may get caught and form deposits in your arteries causing them to narrow. This is how cardiovascular disease and heart disease develop.

Dietary Fat

Dietary fats are those fats that we consume through foods. Fatty acids are components of fat molecules, and they are classified based on the amount of hydrogen they contain. Different kinds of fatty acids result in different production levels of LDL and HDL cholesterol.

Saturated fatty acids come from animal products, including dairy products, and two plant sources, which are coconut and palm oils. Of the three fatty acids, saturated fatty acids result in the greatest production of LDL cholesterol by the liver. There is a misconception that avoiding dietary cholesterol alone will reduce risk for heart disease. However, your own body actually produces most of your blood cholesterol. Only some of it is derived from the food you eat.

But saturated fat, which signals high production levels of LDL cholesterol, is a major contributor to high LDL levels. So avoiding foods high in saturated fat is even more important than avoiding dietary cholesterol. Saturated fats are found in foods that are of animal origin and are solid at room temperature. Think bacon, butter, and cheese.

Polyunsaturated fatty acids, which are found in large amounts in corn, safflower, soybean, sesame, and sunflower oils, result in lower production of both HDL and LDL cholesterol. Unlike saturated fat, polyunsaturated fats are liquid at room temperature.

Trans fatty acids are fats that have received a lot of attention in recent years and rightly so. Trans fats are formed when polyunsaturated fats are altered to behave more like saturated fats. If you see the words "hydrogenated" or "partially hydro-genated," you are dealing with trans fats. The problem with trans fats is that in their effort to make a product that tastes and looks like saturated fats, food manu-facturers have made a product that also behaves like a saturated fat in your body. Trans fatty acids, like saturated fatty acids, will trigger higher production of LDL cholesterol. Margarine and many packaged snack foods like chips, crackers, and cookies are often very high in partially hydrogenated oils.

To avoid trans fats, look for margarine-like spreads such as Promise and Smart Balance, which do not contain trans fatty acids. In fact, these two particular spreads consist of plant stanols, which have been shown to not only keep blood cholesterol from rising—they also help *lower* cholesterol.

Our final class of fatty acids consists of the monounsaturated fatty acids. Think of monounsaturated fatty acids as killing two birds with one stone. They raise HDL cholesterol while lowering LDL cholesterol. Monounsaturated fat is found in olives and olive oil, canola oil, and nuts and nut oils like peanut oil. Avocados and coldwater fish are also high in monounsaturated oil.

Essential Fat

As with amino acids, there are fats that we need but cannot produce ourselves. We must get them from food. The two essential fatty acids are linoleic (omega-6) and linolenic (omega-3) fatty acids. Omega-6 fatty acids are found in vegetable oils (soybean, corn, and safflower). They help lower LDL and total cholesterol but may also lower HDL levels.

You've probably heard a lot about the omega-3 fatty acids found in fish. These fatty acids are very effective at reducing inflammation and may play a role in every-thing from preventing cardiovascular disease, diabetes, cancer, and hypertension to alleviating symptoms of autoimmune diseases. They are necessary for growth and development, particularly of the brain. Hence the saying that fish is "brain food." The omega-3s also help maintain joint and skin health. And for women, they play a role in alleviating those nagging premenstrual symptoms. For the martial artist, of course, the reduction of inflammation due to the demands of training is reason enough to take in enough omega-3s.

Omega-3s are found in abundance in fish and flaxseed. It's still not known exact-ly how much flaxseed we need, but the American Heart Association recommends getting 2–3 servings of fish per week. Salmon, herring, and mackerel have the highest omega-3 content. If that's too fishy for you, you can also get your omega-3s from flaxseed. You can buy flaxseed meal and sprinkle it in smoothies or over cereal. There are also a lot of new products like bread and cereals that are fortified with flaxseed.

Finally, while the jury's still out on this subject, use fish oil supplements with caution. First, the FDA does not regulate these supplements, so you'll need to research quality and content for specific brands. Second, as with any other nutrient, taken in excess, fish oils have detrimental effects, such as interfering with blood clotting and causing internal bleeding. Always check with your doctor before starting supplementing with omega-3s.

Table 1 summarizes the effect the various fatty acids have on the fats circulating in your blood.

Table 1. Effect of Fatty Acids on Blood Lipids

Fatty Acid	Total Cholesterol	LDL	HDL	Triglycerides
Monounsaturated	decrease	decrease	decrease	
Omega-3 (linolenic)	decrease			decrease
Polyunsaturated	decrease	decrease	decrease	
Saturated	increase	increase		
Trans	increase	increase	decrease	

Adapted from Duyff, R.L. 2002

How Much Fat?

For the general public, it's recommended that 30% or less of total daily calories come from fat. Ten percent or less should come from saturated fats. For the lean and mean, however, recommended total fat should account for only 20% total daily calories, with 5% coming from saturated fat. But as always, ratios for optimum health will vary from individual to individual. Later in this book, you'll find examples of appropriate fat portions for various caloric requirements.

CHAPTER 7

Body Composition

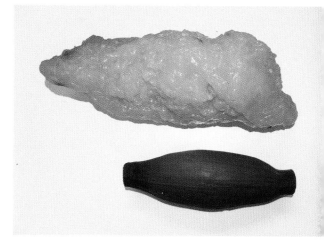

Simulated models of five pounds of fat (top) vs. five pounds of muscle (bottom).

Body Fat

We know that high levels of body fat are associated with a host of health problems, but how can fat hinder athletic performance? Fat is literally an additional burden because, unlike muscle, it's dead weight. Muscle is tissue that enables you to do work. It allows you to move your various body parts—your arms, your legs, your torso. When you throw out a stiff jab, it's muscle that makes that happen. Fat, on the other hand, is just along for the free ride. To make matters worse, fat is less dense than muscle, so it takes up more space. That means you have more surface area causing air friction, which will slow you down.

If your sport requires you to propel those body parts through space—and martial arts do—having more force-producing muscle with less surface area will enhance your performance. And if you're carrying excess baggage around, you can't move those body parts as fast, so you can't produce as much power. Granted, there are some sports where a greater amount of body fat is advantageous. In swimming, for instance, body fat contributes to greater buoyancy. In the martial arts, however, a higher body fat percentage does not yield performance benefits.

Let's be clear, though. You do need some fat. At zero percent body fat, you would die. From a structural point of view, fat helps fill in space and gives structure under your skin. More important to martial artists, fat provides a protective layer around your bones and organs, so you might be more appreciative of that little pad of blubber the next time you take a body shot.

Weight vs. Body Composition

People are obsessed with their weight. Lose weight, gain weight, maintain weight. What is my optimal weight? What can I do to lose weight? Yay, I lost some weight. WEIGHT, weight, WEIGHT, weight, WEIGHT! This preoccupation with the scale has its origins in research that has found people with higher body weight are at increased risk for an array of conditions including cardiovascular disease and diabetes. This may be true for those who are moderately active or sedentary, but it's not the best indicator of health or fitness for very active people. Those just starting exercise programs often complain that since they've started exercising, they've gained weight, not lost it. There are several reasons for this.

First, muscle has higher density than fat and, therefore, weighs much more than fat. The photo on page 51 shows models of 5 pounds of fat and 5 pounds of muscle. Big difference, right? So when dealing with body composition issues, it's better to think about how much space you take up instead of how much you weigh.

The second reason weight is not a good health indicator for athletes is that as you increase exercise and your capacity for exercise, your body adapts by enabling you to store more glycogen. Remember, glycogen is the storage form of clean-burning carbohydrate fuel. Glycogen must be stored with water—more precisely, one molecule of glycogen is stored with 3 molecules of water. And as you'll read in the fluid chapter, 2 cups of water weigh 1 pound, so your hydration status, as well as your glycogen stores, are going to influence your weight.

For these reasons, when assessing active people, we like to use a more accurate measure than weight. Instead, we determine body composition—that is, the percentage of you that is composed of fat versus the percentage of you that is *not* composed of fat, which includes your bones, tendons, organs, and of particular interest to athletes, muscle.

How Is Body Composition Assessed?

There are several methods for assessing body composition, although each has its own limitations and potential pitfalls.

Still considered one of the most accurate methods of body composition testing, hydrostatic weighing is based on the principle that when placed in a water tank, objects of lower density take up more space and, therefore, will displace more water than higher density objects. The problem with hydrostatic weighing, however, is that it is very impractical. It involves thousands of dollars of equipment, not to mention a whole lot of space for a water tank. And unless the technicians are highly skilled, the potential for error outweighs the benefits of using this technique. Subjects often find underwater weighing to be a very unpleasant experience as well. You must completely exhale before submerging yourself. This is the opposite of what we normally do before going underwater! And if you aren't still enough once underwater, you'll have to repeat the test.

Another method of testing body composition is by bioelectrical impedance analysis (BIA). This involves sending an electrical current through the body. Since water efficiently conducts electricity, and muscle consists of a great deal of water, we can expect the current to meet less resistance in a lean subject. Fat, on the other hand, has very little water, and does not conduct electricity well. The current is sent through the subject and then the amount that leaves the subject is measured. The accuracy of this method is improving, although the subject must be sufficiently hydrated. Achieving this level of hydration may be impractical. Any foods with diuretic properties must be avoided and athletes should have a full day of rest prior to the test.

I'm still not sold on BIA. I know of one subject whose foot was immobilized for weeks following foot surgery. We placed her on a $4,000 machine and it measured the resistance through that leg as additional muscle, not fat. We never heard back from the manufacturer on that one. I've also held onto BIA machines and watched my composition drop five percent within two minutes. Now either that machine isn't too accurate or I've discovered a new workout method worth billions.

Dual-Energy-X-Ray Absorptiometry (DEXA) is now considered the gold standard of body composition testing. DEXA provides us with much more detailed information. It gives you information on where body fat *and* muscle are distributed, and since everyone distributes differently, this is very useful information. DEXA works by passing two X-rays through your body and measuring the absorption. This tells us about the density of the material, which is how we determine what type of material it is—bone, muscle, or fat. DEXA is usually used for bone scans. While it is the most accurate method of measuring composition, it's also very expensive. The machine itself can run upwards of $20,000 and for the consumer, a single test will cost a couple hundred dollars. Not too practical or economical if you need to measure your progress weekly, which brings us to the benefits of skinfold calipers.

Skinfold Calipers and "The Pinch"

No, "the pinch" is not the Vulcan grip, so you can relax. We're only measuring the amount of fat we can pinch under your skin. We pick up as much fat as we can pinch and then measure its thickness with a tool called a skinfold caliper. We then plug these numbers into an equation, which yields a prediction of the total body fat percentage. The equations are based on results derived from hydrostatic weighing. Different equations are applied based on sex, age, and number of skinfold sites.

Results from skinfold calipers can be quite accurate if done by a skilled professional. The more skinfold sites measured and the more specific the equation, the better the results. Calipers yield a plus or minus 3% error. And unlike BIA or hydrostatic weighing, they give you an idea of *where* you tend to store your body fat.

Because calipers are so practical and reliable, they are the most widely used tools for assessing body composition. A good pair of calipers can range from $100 to $500. You can also buy cheapie plastic ones under 10 bucks, and some of these are pretty accurate.

I've had several clients do the hydrostatic weighing test and we've come within 2% of their readings with the calipers in each case. That's pretty good, especially when you consider the practicality of calipers and the additional information they provide. Sometimes old school really is better.

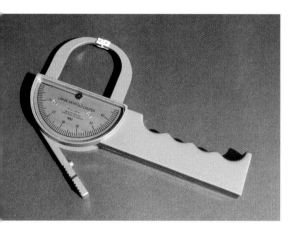

Skinfold calipers are a practical, economical tool for measuring your weekly progress.

Before We Get Hung Up on the Numbers...

Before we delve further into this issue of body composition and body fat percentage, I want to caution you not to become overly preoccupied with your body fat percentage. First, as we've noted, all methods of body fat testing are subject to some degree of error. With calipers, numbers will vary due to factors including the type of caliper and the person doing the pinch (everyone pinches differently). Because of this, your goal body fat percentage should be given as a range, rather than a specific number. A better way of monitoring progress would be to observe *trends* in body composition change. Instead of concentrating on a single number, get your body fat checked regularly (say, once a week) and then see if you are heading in the right direction.

If using calipers, look for millimeters to decrease at each site. Some dietitians don't even bother with the percentage, which at very low percentages can be skewed by the formula used. Instead, they simply take the caliper measurements, and if the numbers start to decrease, then they know they're making progress.

Normal ranges for the general population are 20–25% for women and 15–18% for men. For athletes, the ranges are 10–20% for women and 5–12% for men.

The use of body fat percentage, however, must be exercised with extreme caution. You *can* go too low. Women generally should not go below 12% and men should not dip below 5% unless under very close supervision. Women who have too little fat will stop producing estrogen, putting themselves at risk for osteoporosis. Likewise, men who are too lean may risk a decline in testosterone.

Another word about numbers. A friend of mine, an Olympic athlete, was constantly told to lose weight when she was in high school despite the fact that she was the best player on the team. This is someone who later went all the way to the Olympics—twice! Coaches, unqualified trainers, well-meaning teammates, and friends are not trained to make such recommendations and should leave such advice to registered dietitians and professionals with some background in sports science or sports nutrition.

This same friend told me how the Olympic team members regularly had their body fat checked. They never received individual nutrition counseling and had a grand total of one group session with a dietitian. As a result, these women were not equipped with the information necessary for lowering or maintaining their body fat. They would starve themselves prior to measurements. Then, feeling deprived— and probably unable to fuel their workouts—they would binge afterwards. Some resorted to purging. Not exactly what you want your country's Olympic team to be doing. I relate this story as an example of the misuse of body fat measurements.

The idea behind measuring body fat for athletes is to determine where the athlete performs best. The numbers and ranges don't mean a whole lot if your performance goes down the tubes with it. As in my friend's case—if she was hammering everyone around her, why change anything? You know what they say: "If it ain't broke…"

As with everything else in nutrition, everyone is different. One person may perform best at a higher body fat percentage than another. The numbers and tables are only to get us in the ballpark. More important, you should listen to your body. Ask yourself how you feel at a certain percentage. Are you energized? Fatigued? Do you have enough endurance to go the distance? Are you faster at a certain percentage? Or are you sluggish? Are you excited about your workouts or are you mentally burnt out? Are you catching colds and infections more frequently? At the first sign of decreased performance or immune function, you should consider backing off from aggressively attempting to lower your percentage.

Within my own practice, I've found that once fighters dip too low, their endurance flags. They may have a six-pack but they're unable to go 12 rounds. For this reason, I tend not to let my fighters go below a certain range of body fat percentage. Everyone, of course, operates optimally at a different percentage, so I pay special attention to performance. If they're strong in long sparring sessions, I'm not going to change too much although I might err on the side of keeping their body fat percentage on the higher side. At the very least, we'll take steps to make sure they don't go any lower. And at the first sign that they're gassing out in their workouts, I'll immediately up the calories.

Using the Skinfold Calipers

If you're doing measurements yourself (but note that a few of the sites are not possible to measure on oneself) or on others, here are some guidelines. Again, the test is only as good as the test operator. If you're going to a professional for caliper measurements, you'll want to go to someone who is following similar guidelines for accuracy. If your trainer is not using these checkpoints consistently and methodically, you'll want to go to one who does. I also recommend that you have the same person measure you every time. A good measurer uses the same methods consistently and going to the same person will reduce error due to individual variation.

There are seven sites for skinfold measurements. They are the chest, thigh, abdomen, triceps, suprailium, midaxilla, subscapula, and calf. As with any test, measuring body fat with the skinfold calipers is only as reliable as the test administrator. It's important to follow the same protocol every time, which should include the following steps:

1. Measurements should be made prior to workouts on dry skin. During exercise, fluid shifts to the skin, giving you inflated readings. If skin is not dry, calipers can also easily slip off the site.

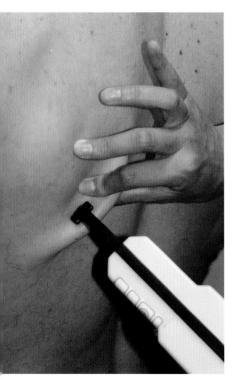

Caliper placement. Calipers should be placed in the middle of the fold.

2. Ask the subject to flex the muscle at the site of measurement and then relax.

3. As the subject relaxes the muscle, grasp the skin at the site with the thumb and the index and middle fingers. You will feel the fat, fold move right into your grasp. If you neglect to have the subject flex and relax, you will most likely grab muscle and fat, and end up with an inflated number.

4. Place the calipers perpendicular to the skinfold. Be sure to place the calipers at the *middle* of the fold, not at the end or where the fold begins and fans out (see photo on page 56). Both will give you inconsistent readings.

5. Let the caliper grip go so that the spring tension on the caliper will stop at the appropriate reading.

6. Take at least three measurements. All should be within 1.0 mm of each other. If they are not, take additional measurements until at least two are within 1.0 mm of each other and then average the two.

7. Measure the same side (left or right) every time.

For very lean subjects, the general landmarks are just that—general landmarks. Since with very lean subjects, it's hard to find something to grab, you'll want to look for slight recesses when they flex. This will be the point of muscle attachment. It will still be in the general area of the landmarks you would normal use, but you will get a more accurate reading measuring at these small recesses because you don't run the risk of pinching muscle as well.

The following are guidelines for specific site measurements.

Chest. Measure the midpoint between the shoulder (anterior axillary line) and nipple. Pinch along the diagonal line between these two points. For subjects who are extremely lean, you will actually pinch at a point where there is a slight recess. This is where the muscle attachment is. It may or may not necessarily be at the midpoint.

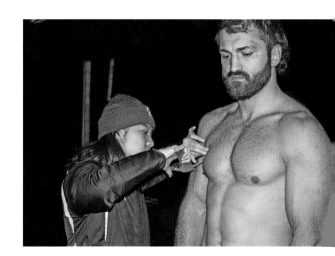

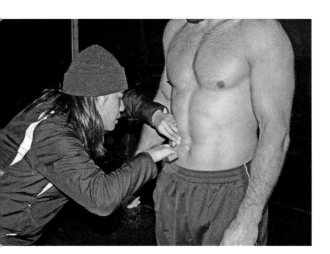

Abdomen. Measure at one inch to the right or left of the belly button (umbilicus) along a vertical line.

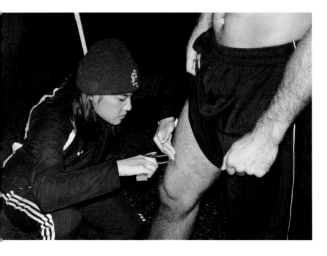

Thigh. Find the midpoint between the hip (at the crease of your leg) and the knee. Measure along a vertical line at the midpoint. Again, when dealing with very lean subjects who may be difficult to pinch, look for the recess at the point of muscle attachment. This is usually below the midpoint.

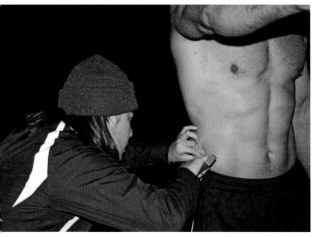

Hip (Suprailiac). Find the top of the subject's hip bone. You can either take this measurement laterally at the top of the bone or just anterior to the crest along a diagonal line.

Triceps. Find the midpoint between the shoulder and elbow (acromion and olecranon processes) along a vertical line. With exceptionally lean subjects, pinch at the point of muscle attachment. As with the thigh site, this is usually below the midpoint.

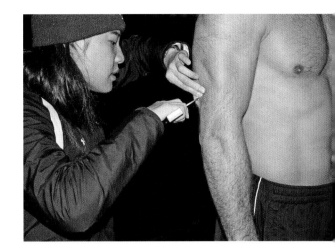

Midaxilla. Find the midaxillary line at the level of the xiphoid process (bottom tip) of the sternum. Pinch along a vertical fold. Lean subjects should actually flex this area before pinching. You'll be able to see the ribs. Pinch along a vertical fold at a point where there is a slight recess between ribs. This point may be slightly below the xiphoid process.

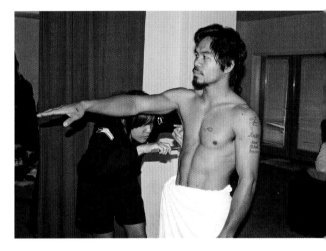

Back (subscapula). Find 1 to 2 cm below the inferior angle of the scapula and measure along a diagonal fold.

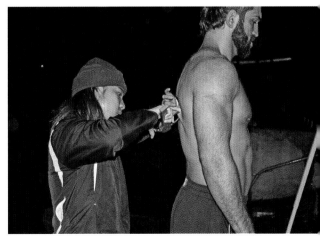

(Photos on pages 56-59: Ariza)

Determining Percentage

There are a gazillion different equations and charts for determining body fat percentage, some more accurate than others. What Works Nutrition Software® uses the Jackson and Pollock formula, which requires three sites. I've used this software for many years now, because it automatically calculates body fat percentage, net weight loss/gain, pounds of fat lost/gained, and pounds of muscle lost/gained. Because as you'll see in the following equations, you can do the math for all this yourself, but software like this makes life so much easier!

If you would like to do things the long way, you can estimate your percentage without the software, however, there are general formulas that determine body composition.

These equations can be quite intricate, so for our purposes know the following denotations:

ΣSKF = sum of skinfolds
Db (g/cc)^a = body density

For women, this is determined by measuring four sites: triceps, abdomen, anterior suprailiac, and thigh.

$$4\Sigma\text{SKF} = \text{triceps} + \text{anterior suprailiac} + \text{abdomen} + \text{thigh}$$

Now determine body density with the following formula:[18]

$$\text{Db (g/cc)}^a = 1.096095 - 0.0006952 \ (4\Sigma\text{SKF}) + 0.0000011 \ (4\Sigma\text{SKF})^2 - 0.0000714 \ (\text{age})$$

For men, the equation involves seven sites:[19]

$$7\Sigma\text{SKF} = \text{chest} + \text{midaxillary} + \text{triceps} + \text{subscapular} + \text{abdomen} + \text{anterior suprailiac} + \text{thigh}$$

And the equation for body density is:

Db (g/cc)^a = 1.112 – 0.00043499 (7∑SKF) + 0.00000055 (7∑SKF)^2 –
    0.00028826 (age)

Now we can convert body density to percentage of body fat with the following equations:[20]

Men %BF = [(4.95/Db) – 4.50] x 100
Women %BF = [(5.01)/Db) – 4.57] x 100

Suppose we have a 27-year-old woman whose measurements are as follows:

triceps = 13.0 mm
anterior suprailiac = 5.0 mm
abdomen = 15.0 mm
thigh = 12.0 mm

The sum of those folds is:

4∑SKF = 13.0 + 5.0 + 15.0 + 12.0 = 45

Now plug this into our formula for body density:

Db (g/cc)^a = 1.096095 – 0.0006952 (45) + 0.0000011 (45)^2 – 0.0000714 (27)
    = 1.096095 – 0.031284 + 0.0022275 – 0.0019278
    = 1.0651107

Now calculate body fat percentage, using the equation for women, which is Women %BF = [(5.01)/Db) – 4.57] x 100.

So:

Women %BF = [(5.01)/ 1.0651107) – 4.57] x 100 = 13.37%

There are, of course, many variations of this formula that are specific to race and age. The formulas used here are for men and women 18–29 years of age. For more specific formulas, check out any physiology or sports medicine text. *Applied Body Composition Assessment* by Heyward and Stolarczyk is a good place to start. Again, it's important not to get too hung up on the actual percentage number. What you're really looking for are trends. Are the millimeters of body fat at each site declining, increasing, or staying where they are?

You can also see that determining body fat from week to week can be quite math intensive. If you plan to chart your progress using percentages to determine muscle and fat gain/loss, then I would suggest using a program like What Works Nutrition Software®. It just makes life a lot easier.

Table 2. Average Body Fat Percentages, Various Athletes

Sport	Male	Female
Ballet dancers	14.50	20.10
Baseball	13.40	n/a
Basketball	9.80	23.90
Distance runners	11.80	17.20
Gymnasts	4.60	19.70
Ice hockey	14.10	n/a
Soccer	6.90	n/a
Swimmers	6.80	18.60
Tennis	16.30	20.30
Volleyball	n/a	23.30
Wrestlers	9.10	n/a

Adapted from McArdle, Katch and Katch 1999

Body Fat Percentage Ranges for Elite Athletes

While there isn't much research on the body composition of martial artists, one study found that elite-level boxers have a body fat percentage of 6.9 + 1.6%. Table 2 shows the average body fat percentages for different athletes. These are not necessarily the optimal ranges for performance, but they give us an idea of how body composition varies from sport to sport. Many of my own clients tend to fall below this range, but this isn't always necessarily desirable.

Losing Weight

Remember we said that an excess of 3500 calories equals one pound of fat. To lose fat, then, we must create an energy deficit. You can do this by restricting calories or exercising to expend more calories or both. Just burning 500 more calories a day will create a 3500-calorie deficit for one week. That means you could lose one pound of fat per week without even restricting food. If you cut calories by 500 and increase exercise so that you expend an additional 500 calories, than you can create a daily deficit of 1000 calories. Therefore, you would lose 2 pounds of fat a week.

As a martial artist, it's not a good idea for you to try losing weight by restricting food alone. You don't want all that training to go out the window, so you need to keep your protein intake up (see Chapter 5) and continue with strength training. Remember muscle is metabolically active tissue. That means it burns calories. Fat is not metabolically active. It makes sense, then, that you would want to have more muscle tissue around. You'll burn more calories just lying in bed if you have more muscle than fat tissue. So if you don't strength train while you're cutting calories, you're making things harder for yourself than they have to be.

Armed with this information, you might say, "Great! If I really cut my calories, then I can lose 20 pounds in a week!" Hold it! You don't want to lose more than 1 to 2 pounds per week. If you crash diet, you will lose muscle as well as fat and water. See Chapter 16 on fluids if you need to be reminded about the dangers of dehydration. Furthermore, you are only fighting a losing battle when you crash diet, because your metabolism will slow down due to muscle loss.

Rapid weight loss and food restriction have been shown to also adversely affect performance and mood. French judoists following a 7-day food restriction exhibited impaired performance in left arm strength and 30-second jumping tests. Micronutrient and carbohydrate intakes were below French recommendations and may have contributed to significant elevation of psychological parameters that included tension, anger, fatigue, and confusion.[21]

In a similar study, boxers required to make weight within a 7-day period shared significant performance decline in a circuit training session and increased tension, fatigue, and anger.[22]

In the following chapter, we'll help you determine energy requirements and avoid negative effects of excessive caloric restriction.

CHAPTER 8

Energy Requirements

Determining Energy Needs

Before you can scientifically alter your body composition, you need a plan, and the first step in building a plan is to determine your energy needs. There are several ways to do this, although they're all rather similar. What we'll be using here is what I've found to be the most practical.

There are four ways in which we expend energy. First, we'll be plugging your current weight into a formula to determine your resting energy expenditure (REE). This is the amount of energy your body needs to function at rest in a 24-hour period. That's you lying in bed asleep, doing nothing except for breathing and maintaining all your other regulatory bodily functions. The second component includes calories for what we call "activities of daily living." Third, we'll also determine additional calories for your present body composition. And, finally, we'll add calories for exercise expenditure.

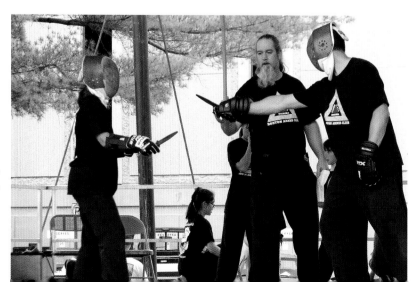

Energy requirements vary greatly from individual to individual.

1. Resting Metabolic Rate (REE)

Did you know that your body spends most of its energy just keeping you alive at rest? The mere regulation of your breathing, digestion, circulation, and body temperature accounts for 60–70% of the calories you require daily. The following revised Harris-Benedict equations are for determining what we call resting energy expenditure (REE), meaning the amount of calories your body requires to function at rest. For men, the equation is:

88.362 + (4.799 x ht) + (13.397 x wt) – (5.677 x age) = REE for males

For women, the equation is:

447.593 + (3.098 x ht) + (9.247 x wt) – (4.330 x age) = REE for females

For both formulas, height is expressed in centimeters, while weight is expressed in kilograms. Let's try an example. Suppose we have a male fighter who is 5'7", weighs 140 pounds and is 30 years old.

First we need to determine his weight in kilograms just as we did in the chapters on carbohydrate and protein. Remember we divide weight in pounds by 2.2 to determine kilograms.

140 ÷ 2.2 = 63.6 kg

We also need to find his height in centimeters. We do this by multiplying his height in inches by 2.54. If our boxer is 5'7", then that's 67 inches.

2.54 x 67 = 170 centimeters

Now we can plug this into our formula.

88.362 + (4.799 x 170cm) + (13.397 x 63.6 kg) – (5.677 x 30)
= 1586 calories

So 1586 calories is what our fighter would need to grow hair, maintain skin health, regulate breathing, etc. while lying around in bed all day. This is what we call his resting energy expenditure (REE). Note that the largest portion of your daily caloric expenditure comes from your REE, not exercise. While still completely necessary, unless you are a professional athlete, your REE accounts for most of the calories you burn every day.

2. Daily Activity

Next, because our fighter did not get to be a fighter by lying around all day, we have to multiply his REE by an activity factor. This estimates how active you are throughout the day *not* including purposeful exercise. This is a somewhat subjective factor that you will have to determine yourself. Are you generally a nervous, fidgety person or mellow and rather calm? Do you have a desk job or are you a construction worker hauling heavy stuff all day? Use Table 3 to help you decide. An activity factor of 1.5 would be for an office worker, while a factor of 2.1 would be for construction worker.

Table 3. Activity Factor Guidelines

		Activity Factor
Very light	Sedentary, bedrest	1.2 - 1.3
Light	No planned activity, office work	1.4 - 1.6
Moderate	Walking, stairclimbing throughout day	1.6 - 1.7
Heavy	Planned vigorous activity	1.9 - 2.1

Adapted from Rosenbloom (Ed.) 2000

Let's say our fighter is rather calm, has an office job, and aside from his training, does not do a lot of strenuous activity. We'll give him an activity factor of 1.4. We take this factor and multiply it by our REE result.

1586 x 1.4 = 2220 calories

Now it's your turn.

1. First we need to determine your weight in kilograms. Divide your weight in pounds by 2.2 to determine kilograms.

   _____ ÷ 2.2 = _____ kg
   (your weight in pounds)

2. We now need to find your height in centimeters. Multiply your height in inches by 2.54.

   _____ x 2.54 = _____ cm
   (your height in inches)

3. Plug this into one of the formulas.

   REE for men:
   88.362 + (4.799 x ht) + (13.397 x wt) − (5.677 x age) = _____ calories

   REE for women:
   447.593 + (3.098 x ht) + (9.247 x wt) − (4.330 x age) = _____ calories

4. Now multiply your answer in step 3 by your activity factor.

3. Determining Energy Expenditure from Exercise

Now it's time to calculate the calories you burn up working out. To do this, we follow these steps:

1. Determine body weight in kilograms. (Body weight in pounds divided by 2.2)
2. Add the number of hours spent engaged in each mode of training.
3. Multiply body weight in kilograms by the number of calories that a particular activity requires per hour and then multiply by the number of hours per week engaged in an activity.
4. Repeat steps 1 through 3 for each activity.
5. Add the total amount of calories burned for all activities.
6. Divide the total by 7. This gives you a daily average of calories spent for exercise.

Table 4 is a list of calories expended per kilogram body weight per hour for activities in which martial artists are often engaged.

Table 4. Exercise and Energy Expenditure

Activity	Calories/kg/hr
Basketball	8.28
Boxing, in ring, general	12.0
Boxing, sparring	9.0
Dance, ballet, modern	6.0
Cycling, leisure	4.0
Cycling, moderate	8.0
Cycling, racing	12.0
Fencing	6.0
Football	9.0
Hockey	8.0
Judo	10.0
Karate	10.0
Kick boxing	10.0
Rock Climbing, ascending	11.0
Rugby	10.0
Running, 5 mph (12 min/mile)	8.0
Running, 6 mph (10 min/mile)	10.0
Running, 7 mph (8.5 min/mile)	11.5
Running, 8 mph (7.5 min/mile)	13.5
Running, 9 mph (6.5 min/mile)	15.0
Running, 10 mph (6 min/mile)	16.0
Running, 10.9 mph (5.5 min/mile)	18.0
Running, stairs	15.0
Soccer	10.0
Squash	12.0
Skipping rope, moderate, general (70 revolutions/min)	10.0
Skipping rope, fast pace (125 revolutions/min)	12.0

Continued

Table 4 (continued)

Activity	Calories/kg/hr
Surfing	3.0
Swimming, freestyle, moderate	8.0
Swimming, freestyle, fast	10.0
Swimming, breast stroke	10.0
Swimming, butterfly	11.0
Swimming, backstroke	8.0
Taekwondo	10.0
Tai Chi	4.0
Tennis, singles	8.0
Tennis, doubles	6.0
Volleyball, general	4.0
Volleyball, beach	8.0
Weightlifting, light to moderate effort	3.0
Weightlifting, power lifting, bodybuilding, vigorous effort	6.0
Wrestling	6.0
Yoga	4.0

Let's walk through an example. Say our boxer has the following weekly training schedule.

Mondays, Wednesdays, and Fridays: ½ hour running at 7 mph, 2 hours boxing training

Tuesdays and Thursdays: ½ hour of wrestling, 2 hours sparring

Saturday: 1 hour of wrestling, ½ hour of rope skipping moderate pace

Remember our fighter weighs 140 pounds, which is 63.6 kilograms.

From the training schedule above, add up the number of hours per week spent in each activity. It shakes out like this:

1.5 hours running at 7 mph
6 hours boxing training

4.0 hours sparring

2 hours wrestling

0.5 hours rope skipping

Now use Table 4 to determine the number of calories required for each activity per kg per hour. Plug that info into the following:

(calories/kg/hour) x (body weight in kg) x (hours spent in activity)

= total calories for activity

So to calculate the number of calories spent running per week for our 63.6 kg fighter:

11.5 calories/kg/hour of **running** x 63.6 kg x 1.5 hours running

= 1097 calories

We then do this for all physical activities for the week:

12.0 calories/kg/hour **boxing** x 63.6 kg x 6.0 hours boxing = 4579 calories

9.0 calories/kg/hour of **sparring** x 63.6 kg x 4.0 hours sparring

= 2290 calories

6.0 calories/kg/hour of **wrestling** x 63.6 kg x 2.0 hours weightlifting

= 763 calories

10.0 calories/kg/hour of **skipping** x 63.6 kg x 0.5 hours skipping

= 318 calories

Now we add the weekly totals of calories required for each activity:

1097	calories for running
4579	calories for boxing training
2290	calories for sparring
763	calories for wrestling
+ 318	calories for skipping
9047	total calories required for one week of exercise

Divide the answer by 7 (because there are 7 days in the week) to determine the number of calories needed for an average day:

> 9047 calories per week ÷ 7 days/week
> = 1292 calories per day for exercise

Skip the Math:
The Easy Way to Determine Exercise Energy Expenditure

If you don't want to be bothered by making all these calculations for your exercise calories, you'll want to pick up a heart rate monitor. We'll get into how to use the heart rate monitor for training purposes in Chapter 11, but monitors can also track the calories you burn during exercise.

You'll still want to incorporate the numbers from your heart rate into a weekly exercise plan and daily nutrition plan. You wouldn't, for example, see that you burned 1200 kcal one day and then try to calculate what you'll be eating on the same day because of that. In my experience, that never works. You'll still want to determine an average number of calories you burn in exercise for the week and then base your *daily* nutrition plan on a daily average of exercise expenditure.

No matter how you do it, once you've calculated your total calories in expended in exercise, simply divide this number by 7 days of the week. This tells you how much energy it takes for you to pay for all of the exercise you did during the week.

All we have to do now is calculate our fighter's total calorie needs for one day. Remember when we multiplied his REE by an activity factor? We just add that result to the number of calories expended per day for exercise.

> (REE x activity factor) + energy required for exercise per day

> 2220 calories + 1292 calories
> = 3512 calories total energy expenditure per day

4. Thermic Effect of Food (TEF)

Muscle is metabolically active tissue. Fat is not. This means that the more muscle and less fat you have, the more calories you burn at rest. You get extra calories, then, based on your body composition! If you know your body fat percentage, use the following table then multiply the factor by your total calories thus far.

Table 5. Thermic Effect of Food Table

Body Fat %, Men	TEF Factor	Body Fat %, Women	TEF Factor
0%	10.00	0%	10.00
15%	10.00	-	-
16%	9.60	-	-
17%	9.20	-	-
18%	8.80	-	-
19%	8.40	-	-
20%	8.00	-	-
21%	7.60	-	-
22%	7.20	22%	10.00
23%	6.80	23%	9.25
24%	6.40	24%	8.50
25%	6.00	25%	7.75
26%	5.60	26%	7.00
27%	5.20	27%	6.25
28%	4.80	28%	5.50
29%	4.40	29%	4.75
30%	4.00	30%	4.00

What Works Nutrition Software®

Say our fighter is 9% body fat. He would get the full 10%. So we multiply his total calories by 10%:

3512 kcal x 10% = 351 kcal

Add this to his total kcal:

3512 kcal + 351 kcal = 3863 kcal

Adapting Your Total Caloric Expenditure for Body Composition Goals

Now that you know what your current caloric expenditure is, realize that this is the number of calories you need to stay at your current body composition. To lose body fat and/or gain muscle, you'll need to alter this number. Here's how.

Losing Body Fat

Remember we said it takes an excess of 3500 calories to produce one pound of fat. Conversely, if we want to lose one pound of fat, we have to create an energy deficit of 3500 calories to lose a pound of fat. Divide that 3500 calories by 7 days of the week and we have a 500-calorie-a-day deficit to lose one pound of fat a week.

To create a deficit, I like to subtract 20% of the total calories, so:

3863 kcal x 20% = 773 kcal

Now subtract this from total calories:

3863 kcal – 773 kcal = 3090 kcal

So for our fighter to lose body fat we would give him a total of 3090 kcal per day by creating a deficit of 773 kcal per day.

Gaining Muscle

Just as adding one pound of fat requires an excess of 3500 calories it also takes about 3500 calories to support one pound of muscle. So if you only want to gain muscle and aren't trying to lose fat, you'll want to eat extra calories each day to gain a pound of muscle each week. Some of those additional calories may come from increased protein needs based on your goals, cross training, etc. We showed you how to calculate those needs in the section on protein. Some of those other extra calories should come from carbohydrate. Remember we explained that carbohydrate is the best fuel source for your muscles, allowing them to do the work that will help you build new lean tissue. The rest of those additional calories can come from fat, as long as fat is still 20% or less of your total caloric intake. Use the meal templates at the end of this chapter as a guideline.

If our fighter wants to gain muscle and doesn't need to lose fat, we could add 500 calories to his total energy expenditure of 3863.

3863 calories + 500 calories for weight gain = 4363 calories

The amount of calories to add for weight gain varies. Again, it's important to have someone assess your body composition, so that adjustments can be made to your diet. If you're gaining muscle and fat, then you're getting too many calories. If you're gaining muscle and losing fat, you're right where you should be. Gaining muscle can be tricky. If you're worried about gaining fat, take your calories up in smaller increments of 250 first. If you don't gain any body fat after the first week and are still having trouble gaining muscle, bump that up to an extra 500 kcal per day.

Macronutrient Puzzle Pieces

Now that you know what your total calories should be, we can start putting a meal plan together for you. Various diets require strict percentages of macronutrients. The Zone Diet employs a 40/30/30 ratio of carbs/protein/fat. Other diets are very drastic—limiting fat to 10% of total calories, for example. But once again, we cannot rely on a one-size-fits-all plan. Everyone is different, with different goals, genes, and activity levels.

In my practice, I use What Works Nutrition® software to determine distribution of the macronutrients. From there, I customize for the individual. To take you through all the formulas behind the software would be beyond the scope of this book, so instead, I've provided templates in 500-calorie increments. Choose the one closest to your caloric needs. Remember, this is merely our starting point. Try this caloric level for one week. Then based on your body composition results, you'll make the necessary modifications, which we'll explain after the next chapter.

Daily 1510 Calorie Meal Plan — Individualized Menu

Especially Formulated For: INITIAL TEMPLATE: **1500** Kcals

Carbohydrate:	142 grams (see percentage of total Calories below)
Protein:	141 grams (see percentage of total Calories below)
Fat:	42 grams (see percentage of total Calories below)

This menu shows how the exchange lists can be used to meet your needs. Use the exchange lists to **plan your own menus.**

MEAL 1 @ 8:00 AM

			# OF	EXCHANGES	CARBS	PROTEIN	FAT	KCALS
2	cups	Cheerios	2	Starches/Breads	30	6	2	
1	cup	1/2% Milk	1	Skim/Non-Fat Milk	12	8	1	
6		Egg whites	3	Very Lean Meat/Substitutes	0	21	3	
0		Apple, raw (2" across or 4oz each)	0	Fruit				
5		Walnut Halves	1	Fat	0	0	5	
				Meal 1 Totals	**42**	**35**	**11**	407

**We DO NOT recommend you exercise on an empty stomach! If you exercise early in the morning, (Boot Camp, Spinn class, running, etc)
SWAP MEALS 1 & 2 so that you have something to eat before working out.**

MEAL 2 @ 11:00 AM

			# OF	EXCHANGES	CARBS	PROTEIN	FAT	KCALS
1/2		Pita pocket bread (6"-8" across)	1	Starches/Breads	15	3	1	
2	oz	Chicken/Turkey, white meat, no skin	2	Very Lean Meat/Substitutes	0	14	2	
				Meal 2 Totals	**15**	**17**	**3**	155

MEAL 3 @ 1:00 PM

			# OF	EXCHANGES	CARBS	PROTEIN	FAT	KCALS
2/3 cup		White or Brown Rice	2	Starches/Breads	30	6	2	
4	oz	Chicken, Turkey, Fish	4	Very Lean Meat/Substitutes	0	28	4	
1	cup	raw OR half as many cooked or steamed	1	Vegetable	5	2	0	
1/2 tsp		Oil (canola, olive)	0.5	Fat	0	0	2.5	
		for a FREE SALAD or used in cooking method		Meal 3 Totals	**35**	**36**	**8.5**	361

MEAL 4 @ 3:45 PM

			# OF	EXCHANGES	CARBS	PROTEIN	FAT	KCALS
1 1/2 sheets		Honey Graham Crkrs 4/sheet	1	Starches/Breads	15	3	1	
1/2 cup		cottage cheese (TJ's 1 1/2% fat)	2	Very Lean Meat/Substitutes	0	14	2	
				Meal 4 Totals	**15**	**17**	**3**	155

MEAL 5 @ 7:00 PM

			# OF	EXCHANGES	CARBS	PROTEIN	FAT	KCALS
2/3 cup		White or Brown Rice	2	Starches/Breads	30	6	2	
4	oz	Tenderloin, Salmon	4	Lean Meat/Substitutes	0	28	12	
1	cup	raw OR half as many cooked or steamed	1	Vegetable	5	2	0	
1/2 Tbsp		Brummel & Brown Spread	0.5	Fat	0	0	2.5	
		over rice and veggies OR see fat list for substitutions		Meal 5 Totals	**35**	**36**	**16.5**	433

Desired Weight: [____] lbs

	CARBS	PROTEIN	FAT
GRAMS FROM EACH CATEGORY:	142	141	42
CALORIES FROM EACH CATEGORY:	568	564	378
PERCENTAGES OF CALORIES	37.6%	37.4%	25.0%
TOTAL MEAL CALORIES	1510	Kcals	

Grams of Protein:

Grams of Carbohydrates:

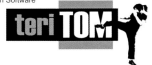

Daily 2010 Calorie Meal Plan — Individualized Menu

Especially Formulated For: INITIAL TEMPLATE: **2000**   Kcals

Carbohydrate:	182 grams (see percentage of total Calories below)
Protein:	190 grams (see percentage of total Calories below)
Fat:	58 grams (see percentage of total Calories below)

This menu shows how the exchange lists can be used to meet your needs. Use the exchange lists to **plan your own menus.**

	MEAL 1 @ 8:00 AM		# OF	EXCHANGES	CARBS	PROTEIN	FAT	KCALS
2	cups	Cheerios	2	Starches/Breads	30	6	2	
1	cup	1/2% Milk	1	Skim/Non-Fat Milk	12	8	1	
6		Egg whites	3	Very Lean Meat/Substitutes	0	21	3	
1		Apple, raw (2" across or 4oz each)	1	Fruit	15	0	0	
5		Walnut Halves	1	Fat	0	0	5	
				Meal 1 Totals	57	35	11	467

We DO NOT recommend you exercise on an empty stomach! If you exercise early in the morning, (Boot Camp, Spinn class, running, etc)
SWAP MEALS 1 & 2 so that you have something to eat before working out.

	MEAL 2 @ 11:00 AM		# OF	EXCHANGES	CARBS	PROTEIN	FAT	KCALS
1/2		Pita pocket bread (6"-8" across)	1	Starches/Breads	15	3	1	
2	oz	Chicken/Turkey, white meat, no skin	2	Very Lean Meat/Substitutes	0	14	2	
				Meal 2 Totals	15	17	3	155

	MEAL 3 @ 1:00 PM		# OF	EXCHANGES	CARBS	PROTEIN	FAT	KCALS
2/3 cup		White or Brown Rice	2	Starches/Breads	30	6	2	
6	oz	Chicken, Turkey, Fish	6	Very Lean Meat/Substitutes	0	42	6	
2	cups	raw OR half as many cooked or steamed	2	Vegetable	10	4	0	
1	tsp	Oil (canola, olive)	1	Fat	0	0	5	
		for a FREE SALAD or used in cooking method		Meal 3 Totals	40	52	13	485

	MEAL 4 @ 3:45 PM		# OF	EXCHANGES	CARBS	PROTEIN	FAT	KCALS
1 1/2 sheets		Honey Graham Crkrs 4/sheet	1	Starches/Breads	15	3	1	
1/2 cup		cottage cheese (TJ's 1 1/2% fat)	2	Very Lean Meat/Substitutes	0	14	2	
				Meal 4 Totals	15	17	3	155

	MEAL 5 @ 7:00 PM		# OF	EXCHANGES	CARBS	PROTEIN	FAT	KCALS
2/3 cup		White or Brown Rice	2	Starches/Breads	30	6	2	
6	oz	Tenderloin, Salmon	6	Lean Meat/Substitutes	0	42	18	
2	cups	raw OR half as many cooked or steamed	2	Vegetable	10	4	0	
1	Tbsp	Brummel & Brown Spread	1	Fat	0	0	5	
		over rice and veggies OR see fat list for substitutions		Meal 5 Totals	40	52	25	593

	MEAL 6 @		# OF	EXCHANGES	CARBS	PROTEIN	FAT	KCALS
1/4 cup		Muesli	1	Starches/Breads	15	3	1	
1/2 cup		cottage cheese (fat free)	2	Very Lean Meat/Substitutes	0	14	2	
				Meal 6 Totals	15	17	3	155

Desired Weight: [ ] lbs

	CARBS	PROTEIN	FAT
GRAMS FROM EACH CATEGORY:	182	190	58
CALORIES FROM EACH CATEGORY:	728	760	522
PERCENTAGES OF CALORIES	36.2%	37.8%	26.0%

TOTAL MEAL CALORIES   2010   Kcals

Grams of Protein:

Grams of Carbohydrates:

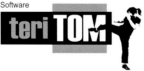

Daily 2516 Calorie Meal Plan — Individualized Menu

Especially Formulated For:		INITIAL TEMPLATE:	**2500** Kcals

Carbohydrate:	227	grams (see percentage of total Calories below)
Protein:	241	grams (see percentage of total Calories below)
Fat:	72	grams (see percentage of total Calories below)

This menu shows how the exchange lists can be used to meet your needs. Use the exchange lists to **plan your own menus.**

MEAL 1 @ 8:00 AM			# OF	EXCHANGES	CARBS	PROTEIN	FAT	KCALS
3	cups	Cheerios	3	Starches/Breads	45	9	3	
1	cup	1/2% Milk	1	Skim/Non-Fat Milk	12	8	1	
8		Egg whites	4	Very Lean Meat/Substitutes	0	28	4	
1		Apple, raw (2" across or 4oz each)	1	Fruit	15	0	0	
7 1/2		Walnut Halves	1.5	Fat	0	0	7.5	
				Meal 1 Totals	**72**	**45**	**15.5**	608

We DO NOT recommend you exercise on an empty stomach! If you exercise early in the morning, (Boot Camp, Spinn class, running, etc) SWAP MEALS 1 & 2 so that you have something to eat before working out.

MEAL 2 @ 11:00 AM			# OF	EXCHANGES	CARBS	PROTEIN	FAT	KCALS
1		Pita pocket bread (6"-8" across)	2	Starches/Breads	30	6	2	
3	oz	Chicken/Turkey, white meat, no skin	3	Very Lean Meat/Substitutes	0	21	3	
				Meal 2 Totals	30	27	5	273

MEAL 3 @ 1:00 PM			# OF	EXCHANGES	CARBS	PROTEIN	FAT	KCALS
2/3 cup		White or Brown Rice	2	Starches/Breads	30	6	2	
7	oz	Chicken, Turkey, Fish	7	Very Lean Meat/Substitutes	0	49	7	
2	cups	raw OR half as many cooked or steamed	2	Vegetable	10	4	0	
1	tsp	Oil (canola, olive)	1	Fat	0	0	5	
		for a FREE SALAD or used in cooking method		Meal 3 Totals	40	59	14	522

MEAL 4 @ 3:45 PM			# OF	EXCHANGES	CARBS	PROTEIN	FAT	KCALS
3	sheets	Honey Graham Crkrs 4/sheet	2	Starches/Breads	30	6	2	
3/4 cup		cottage cheese (TJ's 1 1/2% fat)	3	Very Lean Meat/Substitutes	0	21	3	
				Meal 4 Totals	30	27	5	273

MEAL 5 @ 7:00 PM			# OF	EXCHANGES	CARBS	PROTEIN	FAT	KCALS
2/3 cup		White or Brown Rice	2	Starches/Breads	30	6	2	
7	oz	Tenderloin, Salmon	7	Lean Meat/Substitutes	0	49	21	
2	cups	raw OR half as many cooked or steamed	2	Vegetable	10	4	0	
1	Tbsp	Brummel & Brown Spread	1	Fat	0	0	5	
		over rice and veggies OR see fat list for substitutions		Meal 5 Totals	40	59	28	648

MEAL 6 @			# OF	EXCHANGES	CARBS	PROTEIN	FAT	KCALS
1/4 cup		Muesli	1	Starches/Breads	15	3	1	
3/4 cup		cottage cheese (fat free)	3	Very Lean Meat/Substitutes	0	21	3	
				Meal 6 Totals	15	24	4	192

		CARBS	PROTEIN	FAT
Desired Weight: ___ lbs				
GRAMS FROM EACH CATEGORY:		227	241	72
CALORIES FROM EACH CATEGORY:		908	964	644
PERCENTAGES OF CALORIES		36.1%	38.3%	25.6%
TOTAL MEAL CALORIES		2516	Kcals	

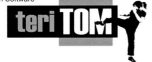

Grams of Protein:

Grams of Carbohydrates:

Daily 3002 Calorie Meal Plan — Individualized Menu

Especially Formulated For:		INITIAL TEMPLATE: **3000** Kcals

Carbohydrate:	280	grams (see percentage of total Calories below)
Protein:	287	grams (see percentage of total Calories below)
Fat:	82	grams (see percentage of total Calories below)

This menu shows how the exchange lists can be used to meet your needs. Use the exchange lists to **plan your own menus.**

MEAL 1 @ 8:00 AM			# OF	EXCHANGES	CARBS	PROTEIN	FAT	KCALS
3	cups	Cheerios	3	Starches/Breads	45	9	3	
1	cup	1/2% Milk	1	Skim/Non-Fat Milk	12	8	1	
8		Egg whites	4	Very Lean Meat/Substitutes	0	28	4	
1		Apple, raw (2" across or 4oz each)	1	Fruit	15	0	0	
7 1/2		Walnut Halves	1.5	Fat	0	0	7.5	
				Meal 1 Totals	**72**	**45**	**15.5**	608

We DO NOT recommend you exercise on an empty stomach! If you exercise early in the morning, (Boot Camp, Spinn class, running, etc) SWAP MEALS 1 & 2 so that you have something to eat before working out.

MEAL 2 @ 11:00 AM			# OF	EXCHANGES	CARBS	PROTEIN	FAT	KCALS
1 1/4		Pita pocket bread (6"-8" across)	2.5	Starches/Breads	37.5	7.5	2.5	
4	oz	Chicken/Turkey, white meat, no skin	4	Very Lean Meat/Substitutes	0	28	4	
				Meal 2 Totals	**37.5**	**35.5**	**6.5**	351

MEAL 3 @ 1:00 PM			# OF	EXCHANGES	CARBS	PROTEIN	FAT	KCALS
1	cup	White or Brown Rice	3	Starches/Breads	45	9	3	
8	oz	Chicken, Turkey, Fish	8	Very Lean Meat/Substitutes	0	56	8	
2	cups	raw OR half as many cooked or steamed	2	Vegetable	10	4	0	
1	tsp	Oil (canola, olive)	1	Fat	0	0	5	
		for a FREE SALAD or used in cooking method		Meal 3 Totals	**55**	**69**	**16**	640

MEAL 4 @ 3:45 PM			# OF	EXCHANGES	CARBS	PROTEIN	FAT	KCALS
3 3/4 sheets		Honey Graham Crkrs 4/sheet	2.5	Starches/Breads	37.5	7.5	2.5	
1	cup	cottage cheese (TJ's 1 1/2% fat)	4	Very Lean Meat/Substitutes	0	28	4	
				Meal 4 Totals	**37.5**	**35.5**	**6.5**	351

MEAL 5 @ 7:00 PM			# OF	EXCHANGES	CARBS	PROTEIN	FAT	KCALS
1	cup	White or Brown Rice	3	Starches/Breads	45	9	3	
8	oz	Tenderloin, Salmon	8	Lean Meat/Substitutes	0	56	24	
2	cups	raw OR half as many cooked or steamed	2	Vegetable	10	4	0	
1	Tbsp	Brummel & Brown Spread	1	Fat	0	0	5	
		over rice and veggies OR see fat list for substitutions		Meal 5 Totals	**55**	**69**	**32**	784

MEAL 6 @			# OF	EXCHANGES	CARBS	PROTEIN	FAT	KCALS
3/8 cup		Muesli	1.5	Starches/Breads	22.5	4.5	1.5	
1	cup	cottage cheese (fat free)	4	Very Lean Meat/Substitutes	0	28	4	
				Meal 6 Totals	**22.5**	**32.5**	**5.5**	270

Desired Weight: _____ lbs	CARBS	PROTEIN	FAT
GRAMS FROM EACH CATEGORY:	280	287	82
CALORIES FROM EACH CATEGORY:	1118	1146	738
PERCENTAGES OF CALORIES	37.2%	38.2%	24.6%
TOTAL MEAL CALORIES	3002	Kcals	

Grams of Protein:

Grams of Carbohydrates:

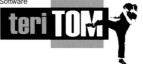

Daily 3562 Calorie Meal Plan — Individualized Menu

Especially Formulated For:

INITIAL TEMPLATE: 3700   Kcals

Carbohydrate:	430	grams (see percentage of total Calories below)
Protein:	269	grams (see percentage of total Calories below)
Fat:	86	grams (see percentage of total Calories below)

This menu shows how the exchange lists can be used to meet your needs. Use the exchange lists to **plan your own menus.**

MEAL 1 @ 8:00 AM			# OF	EXCHANGES	CARBS	PROTEIN	FAT	KCALS
3	cups	Cheerios	3	Starches/Breads	45	9	3	
1	cup	1/2% Milk	1	Skim/Non-Fat Milk	12	8	1	
8		Egg whites	4	Very Lean Meat/Substitutes	0	28	4	
1		Apple, raw (2" across or 4oz each)	1	Fruit	15	0	0	
10		Walnut Halves	2	Fat	0	0	10	
				Meal 1 Totals	72	45	18	630

We DO NOT recommend you exercise on an empty stomach! If you exercise early in the morning, (Boot Camp, Spinn class, running, etc)
SWAP MEALS 1 & 2 so that you have something to eat before working out.

MEAL 2 @ 11:00 AM			# OF	EXCHANGES	CARBS	PROTEIN	FAT	KCALS
1 3/4		Pita pocket bread (6"-8" across)	3.5	Starches/Breads	52.5	10.5	3.5	
4	oz	Chicken/Turkey, white meat, no skin	4	Very Lean Meat/Substitutes	0	28	4	
				Meal 2 Totals	52.5	38.5	7.5	432

MEAL 3 @ 1:00 PM			# OF	EXCHANGES	CARBS	PROTEIN	FAT	KCALS
1 2/3 cups		White or Brown Rice	5	Starches/Breads	75	15	5	
5	oz	Chicken, Turkey, Fish	5	Very Lean Meat/Substitutes	0	35	5	
2	cups	raw OR half as many cooked or steamed	2	Vegetable	10	4	0	
1 1/2 tsp		Oil (canola, olive)	1.5	Fat	0	0	7.5	
		for a FREE SALAD or used in cooking method		Meal 3 Totals	100	54	17.5	774

MEAL 4 @ 3:45 PM			# OF	EXCHANGES	CARBS	PROTEIN	FAT	KCALS
5 1/4 sheets		Honey Graham Crkrs 4/sheet	3.5	Starches/Breads	52.5	10.5	3.5	
1	cup	cottage cheese (TJ's 1 1/2% fat)	4	Very Lean Meat/Substitutes	0	28	4	
				Meal 4 Totals	52.5	38.5	7.5	432

MEAL 5 @ 7:00 PM			# OF	EXCHANGES	CARBS	PROTEIN	FAT	KCALS
1 2/3 cups		White or Brown Rice	5	Starches/Breads	75	15	5	
5	oz	Tenderloin, Salmon	5	Lean Meat/Substitutes	0	35	15	
2	cups	raw OR half as many cooked or steamed	2	Vegetable	10	4	0	
1 1/2 Tbsp		Brummel & Brown Spread	1.5	Fat	0	0	7.5	
		over rice and veggies OR see fat list for substitutions		Meal 5 Totals	100	54	27.5	864

MEAL 6 @			# OF	EXCHANGES	CARBS	PROTEIN	FAT	KCALS
7/8 cup		Muesli	3.5	Starches/Breads	52.5	10.5	3.5	
1	cup	cottage cheese (fat free)	4	Very Lean Meat/Substitutes	0	28	4	
				Meal 6 Totals	52.5	38.5	7.5	432

Desired Weight: _____ lbs

	CARBS	PROTEIN	FAT
GRAMS FROM EACH CATEGORY:	430	269	86
CALORIES FROM EACH CATEGORY:	1718	1074	770
PERCENTAGES OF CALORIES	48.2%	30.2%	21.6%
TOTAL MEAL CALORIES	3562	Kcals	

Grams of Protein:

Grams of Carbohydrates:

© 2000-2006 Lucho Crisalle, RD

What Works™ Nutrition Software

Release 7i-ADULT-0105

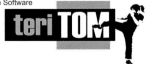

Daily 4011 Calorie Meal Plan — Individualized Menu

Especially Formulated For: INITIAL TEMPLATE: **4200** Kcals

Carbohydrate:	484 grams (see percentage of total Calories below)
Protein:	302 grams (see percentage of total Calories below)
Fat:	97 grams (see percentage of total Calories below)

This menu shows how the exchange lists can be used to meet your needs. Use the exchange lists to ***plan your own menus.***

MEAL 1 @ 8:00 AM			# OF	EXCHANGES	CARBS	PROTEIN	FAT	KCALS
4	cups	Cheerios	4	Starches/Breads	60	12	4	
2	cups	1/2% Milk	2	Skim/Non-Fat Milk	24	16	2	
8		Egg whites	4	Very Lean Meat/Substitutes	0	28	4	
2		Apple, raw (2" across or 4oz each)	2	Fruit	30	0	0	
10		Walnut Halves	2	Fat	0	0	10	
				Meal 1 Totals	114	56	20	860

We DO NOT recommend you exercise on an empty stomach! If you exercise early in the morning, (Boot Camp, Spinn class, running, etc)
SWAP MEALS 1 & 2 so that you have something to eat before working out.

MEAL 2 @ 11:00 AM		# OF	EXCHANGES	CARBS	PROTEIN	FAT	KCALS
1 1/2	Pita pocket bread (6"-8" across)	3	Starches/Breads	45	9	3	
4 1/2 oz	Chicken/Turkey, white meat, no skin	4.5	Very Lean Meat/Substitutes	0	31.5	4.5	
			Meal 2 Totals	45	40.5	7.5	410

MEAL 3 @ 1:00 PM		# OF	EXCHANGES	CARBS	PROTEIN	FAT	KCALS
1 2/3 cups	White or Brown Rice	5	Starches/Breads	75	15	5	
6 oz	Chicken, Turkey, Fish	6	Very Lean Meat/Substitutes	0	42	6	
2 1/2 cups	raw OR half as many cooked or steamed	2.5	Vegetable	12.5	5	0	
2 tsp	Oil (canola, olive)	2	Fat	0	0	10	
	for a FREE SALAD or used in cooking method		Meal 3 Totals	117.5	62	21	907

MEAL 4 @ 3:45 PM		# OF	EXCHANGES	CARBS	PROTEIN	FAT	KCALS
4 1/2 sheets	Honey Graham Crkrs 4/sheet	3	Starches/Breads	45	9	3	
1 1/8 cups	cottage cheese (TJ's 1 1/2% fat)	4.5	Very Lean Meat/Substitutes	0	31.5	4.5	
			Meal 4 Totals	45	40.5	7.5	410

MEAL 5 @ 7:00 PM		# OF	EXCHANGES	CARBS	PROTEIN	FAT	KCALS
1 2/3 cups	White or Brown Rice	5	Starches/Breads	75	15	5	
6 oz	Tenderloin, Salmon	6	Lean Meat/Substitutes	0	42	18	
2 1/2 cups	raw OR half as many cooked or steamed	2.5	Vegetable	12.5	5	0	
2 Tbsp	Brummel & Brown Spread	2	Fat	0	0	10	
	over rice and veggies OR see fat list for substitutions		Meal 5 Totals	117.5	62	33	1015

MEAL 6 @		# OF	EXCHANGES	CARBS	PROTEIN	FAT	KCALS
3/4 cup	Muesli	3	Starches/Breads	45	9	3	
1 1/8 cups	cottage cheese (fat free)	4.5	Very Lean Meat/Substitutes	0	31.5	4.5	
			Meal 6 Totals	45	40.5	7.5	410

Desired Weight: _____ lbs

	CARBS	PROTEIN	FAT
GRAMS FROM EACH CATEGORY:	484	302	97
CALORIES FROM EACH CATEGORY:	1936	1206	869
PERCENTAGES OF CALORIES	48.3%	30.1%	21.7%
TOTAL MEAL CALORIES	4011	Kcals	

Grams of Protein:

Grams of Carbohydrates:

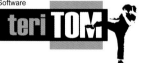

Daily 4499 Calorie Meal Plan — Individualized Menu

Especially Formulated For:	INITIAL TEMPLATE:	**5000** Kcals

Carbohydrate:	564	grams (see percentage of total Calories below)
Protein:	329	grams (see percentage of total Calories below)
Fat:	103	grams (see percentage of total Calories below)

This menu shows how the exchange lists can be used to meet your needs. Use the exchange lists to **plan your own menus.**

MEAL 1 @ 8:00 AM			# OF	EXCHANGES	CARBS	PROTEIN	FAT	KCALS
4	cups	Cheerios	4	Starches/Breads	60	12	4	
2	cups	1/2% Milk	2	Skim/Non-Fat Milk	24	16	2	
8		Egg whites	4	Very Lean Meat/Substitutes	0	28	4	
2		Apple, raw (2" across or 4oz each)	2	Fruit	30	0	0	
10		Walnut Halves	2	Fat	0	0	10	
				Meal 1 Totals	114	56	20	860

**We DO NOT recommend you exercise on an empty stomach! If you exercise early in the morning, (Boot Camp, Spinn class, running, etc)
SWAP MEALS 1 & 2 so that you have something to eat before working out.**

MEAL 2 @ 11:00 AM			# OF	EXCHANGES	CARBS	PROTEIN	FAT	KCALS
2		Pita pocket bread (6"-8" across)	4	Starches/Breads	60	12	4	
5	oz	Chicken/Turkey, white meat, no skin	5	Very Lean Meat/Substitutes	0	35	5	
				Meal 2 Totals	60	47	9	509

MEAL 3 @ 1:00 PM			# OF	EXCHANGES	CARBS	PROTEIN	FAT	KCALS
2	cups	White or Brown Rice	6	Starches/Breads	90	18	6	
6	oz	Chicken, Turkey, Fish	6	Very Lean Meat/Substitutes	0	42	6	
3	cups	raw OR half as many cooked or steamed	3	Vegetable	15	6	0	
2	tsp	Oil (canola, olive)	2	Fat	0	0	10	
		for a FREE SALAD or used in cooking method		Meal 3 Totals	135	66	22	1002

MEAL 4 @ 3:45 PM			# OF	EXCHANGES	CARBS	PROTEIN	FAT	KCALS
6	sheets	Honey Graham Crkrs 4/sheet	4	Starches/Breads	60	12	4	
1 1/4	cups	cottage cheese (TJ's 1 1/2% fat)	5	Very Lean Meat/Substitutes	0	35	5	
				Meal 4 Totals	60	47	9	509

MEAL 5 @ 7:00 PM			# OF	EXCHANGES	CARBS	PROTEIN	FAT	KCALS
2	cups	White or Brown Rice	6	Starches/Breads	90	18	6	
6	oz	Tenderloin, Salmon	6	Lean Meat/Substitutes	0	42	18	
3	cups	raw OR half as many cooked or steamed	3	Vegetable	15	6	0	
2	Tbsp	Brummel & Brown Spread	2	Fat	0	0	10	
		over rice and veggies OR see fat list for substitutions		Meal 5 Totals	135	66	34	1110

MEAL 6 @			# OF	EXCHANGES	CARBS	PROTEIN	FAT	KCALS
1	cup	Muesli	4	Starches/Breads	60	12	4	
1 1/4	cups	cottage cheese (fat free)	5	Very Lean Meat/Substitutes	0	35	5	
				Meal 6 Totals	60	47	9	509

		CARBS	PROTEIN	FAT
Desired Weight: _____ lbs				
GRAMS FROM EACH CATEGORY:		564	329	103
CALORIES FROM EACH CATEGORY:		2256	1316	927
PERCENTAGES OF CALORIES		50.1%	29.3%	20.6%
TOTAL MEAL CALORIES		4499	Kcals	

Grams of Protein:

Grams of Carbohydrates:

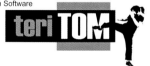

Daily 5004 Calorie Meal Plan — Individualized Menu

Especially Formulated For: INITIAL TEMPLATE: **5000** Kcals

Carbohydrate:	609 grams (see percentage of total Calories below)
Protein:	373 grams (see percentage of total Calories below)
Fat:	120 grams (see percentage of total Calories below)

This menu shows how the exchange lists can be used to meet your needs. Use the exchange lists to **plan your own menus.**

MEAL 1 @ 8:00 AM		# OF	EXCHANGES	CARBS	PROTEIN	FAT	KCALS
5	cups	Cheerios	5	Starches/Breads	**75**	15	5	
2	cups	1/2% Milk	2	Skim/Non-Fat Milk	24	16	2	
8		Egg whites	4	Very Lean Meat/Substitutes	0	**28**	4	
2		Apple, raw (2" across or 4oz each)	2	Fruit	30	0	0	
12 1/2		Walnut Halves	2.5	Fat	0	0	**12.5**	
				Meal 1 Totals	**129**	**59**	**23.5**	964

We DO NOT recommend you exercise on an empty stomach! If you exercise early in the morning, (Boot Camp, Spinn class, running, etc)
SWAP MEALS 1 & 2 so that you have something to eat before working out.

MEAL 2 @ 11:00 AM		# OF	EXCHANGES	CARBS	PROTEIN	FAT	KCALS
2 1/2		Pita pocket bread (6"-8" across)	5	Starches/Breads	**75**	15	5	
5	oz	Chicken/Turkey, white meat, no skin	5	Very Lean Meat/Substitutes	0	**35**	5	
				Meal 2 Totals	**75**	**50**	**10**	590

MEAL 3 @ 1:00 PM		# OF	EXCHANGES	CARBS	PROTEIN	FAT	KCALS
2	cups	White or Brown Rice	6	Starches/Breads	**90**	18	6	
8	oz	Chicken, Turkey, Fish	8	Very Lean Meat/Substitutes	0	**56**	8	
3	cups	raw OR half as many cooked or steamed	3	Vegetable	15	6	0	
2	tsp	Oil (canola, olive)	2	Fat	0	0	**10**	
		for a FREE SALAD or used in cooking method		Meal 3 Totals	**135**	**80**	**24**	1076

MEAL 4 @ 3:45 PM		# OF	EXCHANGES	CARBS	PROTEIN	FAT	KCALS
7 1/2 sheets		Honey Graham Crkrs 4/sheet	5	Starches/Breads	**75**	15	5	
1 1/4 cups		cottage cheese (TJ's 1 1/2% fat)	5	Very Lean Meat/Substitutes	0	**35**	5	
				Meal 4 Totals	**75**	**50**	**10**	590

MEAL 5 @ 7:00 PM		# OF	EXCHANGES	CARBS	PROTEIN	FAT	KCALS
2	cups	White or Brown Rice	6	Starches/Breads	**90**	18	6	
9	oz	Tenderloin, Salmon	9	Lean Meat/Substitutes	0	**63**	27	
3	cups	raw OR half as many cooked or steamed	3	Vegetable	15	6	0	
2	Tbsp	Brummel & Brown Spread	2	Fat	0	0	**10**	
		over rice and veggies OR see fat list for substitutions		Meal 5 Totals	**135**	**87**	**43**	1275

MEAL 6 @		# OF	EXCHANGES	CARBS	PROTEIN	FAT	KCALS
1	cup	Muesli	4	Starches/Breads	**60**	12	4	
1 1/4 cups		cottage cheese (fat free)	5	Very Lean Meat/Substitutes	0	**35**	5	
				Meal 6 Totals	**60**	**47**	**9**	509

Desired Weight: [   ] lbs

What Works™ Nutrition Software

Release 7i-ADULT-0105

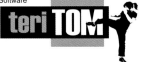

	CARBS	PROTEIN	FAT
GRAMS FROM EACH CATEGORY:	609	373	120
CALORIES FROM EACH CATEGORY:	2436	1492	1076
PERCENTAGES OF CALORIES	48.7%	29.8%	21.5%
TOTAL MEAL CALORIES	5004		Kcals

Grams of Protein:

Grams of Carbohydrates:

CHAPTER 9

The Exchange System

Exchange Lists

The easiest way to organize your meal plan is to understand the exchange system. I tell my clients that the exchange system is just a fancy way of saying "standardizing quantities of food." It enables us to track what you're eating.

Why is this important to you as a martial artist? Because your safety—back in the day, it was your *life*—depends on your performance, and your performance improvement depends on following repeatable, quantifiable methods. Following this procedure consistently yields known, measurable results. Just as you would with a baking recipe or chemistry lab experiment, you need to measure the ingredients and materials. Otherwise, the results are meaningless. The exchange system allows us to measure the ingredients contributing to your body composition and athletic performance.

The American Diabetes Association originally developed the exchange system so diabetics could determine their carbohydrate intake and balance their diets with ease and flexibility. The system consists of a set of food lists. Foods are listed together based on their nutrition content, so foods with equivalent amounts of carbohydrate, protein, and fat are grouped together. The lists include the following categories: starches, fruit, milk, other carbohydrates, vegetables, fat, and meat and meat substitutes. Foods within a single list are interchangeable with any other food on that same list. For example, one slice of bread is equivalent to ½ cup of pasta, because both provide approximately 15 grams of carbohydrate, 3 grams of protein, and 0–1 grams of fat. Therefore, these items are both found on the starch list.

Foods are placed on a particular list based on the nutrition constituent that is most prevalent in that food. So while beans may be high in protein, they are even higher in carbohydrate. A half cup of black beans consists of 8 grams of protein and 21 grams of carbohydrate. The carbohydrate content is almost 3 times that of protein. For this reason, beans are placed on the starch/bread list.

The starch, fruit, milk, and vegetable lists all fall under the carbohydrate category. Starch, fruit, and milk have approximately the same amount of carbohydrate and may be exchanged for each other. So if you are not a regular milk drinker but decide to have a cup once in awhile, on those days you would count an exchange of milk as one of your starch exchanges.

Table 6 shows the nutritional content of items on each of the exchange lists.

Table 6. Macronutrient Content of Exchange Lists

List	Carbohydrate (g)	Protein (g)	Fat (g)	Calories
Starch	15	3	0–1	80
Fruit	15	-	-	60
Milk				
Fat-Free	12	8	0–3	90
Reduced-Fat	12	8	5	120
Whole	12	8	8	150
Other Carbohydrates	15	varies	varies	varies
Vegetables	5	2	-	25
Meat and Meat Substitutes				
Very Lean	-	7	0-1	35
Lean	-	7	3	55
Medium Fat	-	7	5	75
High Fat	-	7	8	100
Fat	-	-	5	45

American Dietetic Association

Serving vs. Exchange

You may have noticed that the nutrition labels on food packages show serving sizes and nutrition information per serving. It is important to note that this serving size is not standardized and is determined by food companies. So one company may make a small bagel that consists of 15 grams of carbohydrate. They may call this one serving. Another company may make a larger bagel that is 45 grams of carbohydrate but may also call this one serving, even though you would be getting 3 times the calories compared to the small bagel.

To clear up some of the confusion, the American Diabetes Association and the American Dietetic Association came up with a system that would provide some standardization. Since the word "serving" had already been taken, they decided to use the word "exchange." As you know, one carbohydrate exchange provides 15 grams of carbohydrate. So that small bagel would be one exchange. The large bagel, however, contains 45 grams of carbohydrate. We divide this number by 15 to find that this large bagel is equivalent to 3 exchanges.

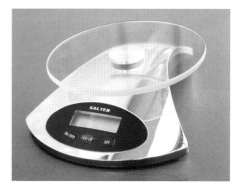

Tools like food scales and measuring cups enable you to accurately track your food intake.

Using the Exchanges

On a single exchange list the nutrition content of any item *in the appropriate portion size* is equivalent to the nutrition content of any other item on that list *in the appropriate portion size.*

So from the fat list (on page 96), 6 almonds are equivalent to 1 teaspoon of olive oil. Both provide 5 grams of fat and 45 calories. But if I were to have 18 almonds instead of 6, I'd be getting 15 grams of fat and 135 calories. That's a big difference. In another example, ½ cup of orange juice is equivalent to 15 grams of carbohydrate and 60 calories. If I were to drink a whole cup, however, I would be getting twice the calories. If I fail to account for this extra 15 grams of carbohydrate, then I will have a tough time making progress toward my body composition goals. Controlling your portion sizes can make or break you.

In the beginning it's important to use measuring cups and to weigh your food. Reading labels will also help you monitor your intake. It may seem a little tedious at first, but after awhile you will become better at approximating and memorizing portion sizes.

Armed with the exchange lists, we can now use them with the calorie templates in the previous chapter. Let's take our daily 2,000 calorie meal plan, as an example. The middle column will tell you the number of exchanges. So for breakfast, there are 2 starch/bread exchanges. Using our starch/bread list, we know one exchange is ½ English muffin. Since we get two exchanges, we multiply by two—we get the whole muffin. Or if we were to choose Special K, we know 1 cup is equal to one exchange. We get 2 exchanges, so we get 2 cups. You can also mix and match— 1 cup of Special K and ½ English muffin—whatever gets you two exchanges.

How to Measure

You can quantify your intake either by volume, weight, or size of an item. Liquids are generally measured by volume because this is easier to eyeball when you don't have a food scale available. Weight, however, is also an acceptable measure. Grains are also usually listed by volume and fruits by size for the same reason—they're easier to eyeball when you're eating out. Proteins like meat and poultry are best measured by weight (after cooking) but since this is not always practical, when I'm out, I use the approximation that 3 oz of cooked chicken, turkey, fish, or beef is about the size of a deck of cards. So if my plan allows for 6 very lean meat exchanges, I would have a serving size of turkey about the size of 2 decks of cards. If I'm home, though, I'll weigh the portion to be more accurate.

Hit the Bold Numbers

If you have the nutrition label for an item, you can also use your daily meal plan (see the plans on pages 75–82) to determine your portion size. Say you have a box of cereal and you're not sure what your portion size should be. Since you know cereal is in the starch/bread category, on your meal plan—for example, let's say it's the 1500-calorie plan on page 75—read across from the starch/bread line to the columns on the right. You'll see the number 30 in bold. It's in the carbs column. That's your number. Try to hit a portion size that gets you as close to 30 g of carbs as possible.

Say you have a protein powder you're not sure about. You know it's in the very lean meat/substitute category. Read across from the very lean meat/substitute line and you'll see the number 21 in bold. Your portion size should get you 21 g of protein.

If you have a meal replacement, like a shake or bar, or an item where all the macronutrients are combined, like a frozen dinner or a burrito, then look for the meal totals. These are located in bold at the bottom of each meal breakdown.

Don't drive yourself too crazy trying to hit the other numbers exactly. If you're off a few grams here or there, it won't kill you. Just be sure to hit the bold numbers for the appropriate food category.

More Lists

The exchange lists in this book come from the What Works Nutrition® database. They are by no means comprehensive lists but should give you an idea of how the system works. Also note that numbers vary considerably from brand to brand, so if you have the nutrition label for something—and most foods do—be sure to use the label, as it is specific to the product.

You can also look up more comprehensive exchange lists online, at sites including www.nhlbi.nih.gov, www.diabetes.org and www.mayoclinic.com. There are also a number of exchange list and food count books available. And once you know the constituents of each kind of exchange, you can also calculate from any nutrition label what the exchanges are.

The Exchange Lists
Starch Lists

1 starch exchange (15 g CHO, 3 g protein, 0–1 g fat, 80 calories)

Cereals		
Bran Cereal	½	cup
Cheerios	1	cup
Corn Chex	½	cup
Corn Flakes	½	cup
Cream of Rice	½	cup
Cream of Wheat	½	cup
Fiber One	¼	cup
Fruit & Fibre (Harvest Medley)	⅓	cup
Go Lean	⅜	cup
Granola	¼	cup
Grape Nuts	⅛	cup
HeriTage Cereal	½	cup
Kasha	½	cup
Kashi Breakfast Pilaf	¼	cup
Kashi Honey Puffed	⅗	cup
Kellogg's Special K	1	cup
Life Cereal	½	cup
Muesli	¼	cup

Continued

Cereals (continued)		
Oatmeal, cooked	½	cup
Post Shredded Wheat n' Bran	½	cup
Puffed Wheat Cereal	1 ½	cup
Quaker Oatmeal Squares	⅓	cup
Raisin Bran	⅓	cup
Rice Chex	½	cup
Rice Crispies	¾	cup
Shredded Wheat	½	cup
Smart Start	⅓	cup
Wheat Chex	½	cup
Wheat Germ	3	Tbsp

Other Breakfast Foods	
Pancakes, 4 inches across	2
Waffles, 4½ inch square	1

White or Brown Rice	⅓	cup
Couscous	⅓	cup
Bulgur	½	cup

Pasta		
Pasta, cooked (most types although varies by brand/manufacturer)	½	cup
Dumplings or gnocchi, steamed (small)	2	

Breads		
Bagel	1	oz
English Muffin	½	
Muffins (most)	⅓	muffin
Bread (most types)	1	slice
Ezekiel 4:9 Bread	1	slice
Lite Bread	2	slices
Northridge Orowheat	1 ½	slices
Orowheat Health Nut Bread	⁵/₆	slice
Orowheat Seven Grain Bread	1 ⅓	slice
Raisin Bread	⁵/₆	slice

Continued

Breads (continued)		
Pita pocket bread (6"–8" across)	½	
Roll, small	1	roll
Sandwich/Hamburger bun	½	bun
Hot Dog bun	½	bun
Tortilla (6" corn or 8" flour)	1	

Crackers and Cookies		
Animal Crackers	4	
Breton Crackers	5 ½	crackers
Breton Sesame Crackers	6 ½	crackers
Cabaret Crackers	5	crackers
Graham Crackers, low-fat 4/sheet	1.5	sheet
Graham Crackers, 4/sheet	1.5	sheet
Gingersnaps	3	
Triscuits	5	
Matzo crackers	7	crackers
Popcorn (plain, popped)	3	cups
Pretzels	¾	oz
Rice Cakes (varies with brand)	2	
Ritz Crackers	$6 \frac{2}{3}$	
Ry Krisp crackers	3	crackers
Stoned Wheat Thins	3	

Starchy Vegetables		
Cooked Beans (pinto, garbanzo, etc.)	$\frac{1}{3}$	cup
Corn meal	2	tbsp
Corn on the cob (6" each)	1	
Corn	½	cup
Mixed vegetables w/corn, peas, or pasta	1	cup
Peas (green)	½	cup
Plantain (green mature), cooked	$\frac{1}{3}$	cup
Potato, baked, boiled or steamed	3	oz
Potato, mashed	½	cup
Squash (winter: acorn, hubbard, pumpkin)	1	cup
Yam or sweet potato	2	oz

Legumes = 1 Starch plus 1 Very Lean Meat Exchange		
Black-eyed Peas	½	cup
Garbanzo Beans	½	cup
Kidney Beans	½	cup
Lentils	½	cup
Lima Beans	²/₃	cup
Pinto Beans	½	cup
Split Peas	½	cup
White Beans	½	cup

Fruit Lists

1 fruit exchange (15 g CHO, 0 g protein, 0 g fat, 60 calories)

Fruits		
Apple, raw (2" across or 4 oz each)	1	
Applesauce, no sugar added	½	cup
Apples, dried	4	rings
Apricots, fresh (1.3 oz each)	4	whole
Apricots, dried	8	halves
Apricots, canned	½	cup
Banana (9" long)	½	
Berries (blackberries, blueberries)	¾	cup
Berries (raspberries, boysenberries)	1	cup
Cantaloupe or honeydew melon (cubed)	1	cup
Cherries	12	
Cherries, canned or jarred	½	cup
Dates	3	
Figs, fresh (medium)	2	
Figs, fresh (large)	1 ½	
Figs, dried	1 ½	
Fruit cocktail	½	cup
Grapefruit (large)	½	
Grapefruit sections, canned	¾	cup
Grapes (small)	15	
Grapes (large)	10	

Continued

Fruit (continued)		
Kiwi (3½ oz each)	1	
Mandarin oranges, canned	½	cup
Mango (small)	½	
Nectarine, small (5 oz each)	1	
Orange (2½″ across)	1	
Papaya	1	cup
Peach medium, fresh (6 oz each)	1	
Peaches, canned	½	cup
Pear, large, fresh (4 oz each)	½	
Pears, canned	½	cup
Pineapple, fresh	¾	cup
Pineapple, canned	½	cup
Plums, raw (2″ across or 5 oz each)	2	
Plums, canned	½	cup
Prunes, dried	2	
Raisins	2	tbsp
Strawberries, fresh, whole	1 ¼	cup
Tangerines, small (8 oz each)	2	
Watermelon	1 ¼	cup

Fruit Juice		
Apple juice/cider	½	cup
Cranberry juice cocktail	$^1/_3$	cup
Cranberry juice cocktail, reduced cal.	1	cup
Fruit juice blends	$^1/_3$	cup
Grape juice	$^1/_3$	cup
Grapefruit juice	½	cup
Orange juice	½	cup
Pineapple juice	½	cup
Prune juice	$^1/_3$	cup

Milk Lists

Fat-Free Milk

1 fat-free milk exchange (12 g CHO, 8 g protein, 0–3 g fat, 90 calories)

Skim Milk (fat free)	1	cup
½% Milk	1	cup
1% Milk	1	cup
Fat Free or Low Fat Buttermilk	1	cup
Evaporated Fat Free Milk	½	cup
Fat Free Dry Milk	⅓	cup
Plain Nonfat Yogurt	¾	cup
Non/Low Fat Fruit-Flavored Yogurt with aspartame	1	cup

Reduced Fat Milk

1 reduced fat milk exchange (12 g CHO, 8 g protein, 5 g fat, 120 calories)

Soy milk	1	cup
2% milk	1	cup
Plain Low Fat Yogurt	¾	cup
Sweet Acidophilus Milk	1	cup

Whole Milk

1 reduced fat milk exchange (12 g CHO, 8 g protein, 8 g fat, 150 calories)

Whole (3%) Milk	1	cup
Evaporated Whole Milk	½	cup
Plain Yogurt	¾	cup

Vegetable Lists

1 vegetable exchange (5 g CHO, 2 g protein, 0 g fat, 25 calories)

Artichoke	½	cup
Artichoke Hearts	½	cup
Beans (green, wax, snap), raw	1	cup
Beans (green, wax, snap), cooked	½	cup
Bean sprouts, raw	1	cup
Beets, raw	1	cup

Continued

Vegetable (continued)		
Beets, cooked	½	cup
Broccoli, raw	1	cup
Broccoli, cooked	½	cup
Cabbage, raw	1	cup
Cabbage, cooked	½	cup
Carrots, raw	1	cup
Carrots, cooked	½	cup
Eggplant, raw	1	cup
Eggplant, cooked	½	cup
Greens, raw	1	cup
Greens, cooked	½	cup
Jicama, raw	1	cup
Jicama, cooked	½	cup
Mushrooms raw	1	cup
Mushrooms, cooked	½	cup
Okra, raw	1	cup
Okra, cooked	½	cup
Peppers, raw	1	cup
Peppers, cooked	½	cup
Sauerkraut	½	cup
Spaghetti Sauce	½	cup
Squash, raw	1	cup
Squash, cooked	½	cup
Vegetable juices	½	cup
Water chestnuts	½	cup

Meat and Meat Substitute Lists
Very Lean Meats and Meat Substitutes

1 very lean meat exchange (0 CHO, 7 g protein, 0 g fat, 35 calories)

Poultry (cooked)		
Chicken, Turkey, Fish	1	oz
Chicken/Turkey, white meat (no skin)	1	oz
Cornish hen (no skin)	1	oz

Fish and Shellfish		
Fresh or frozen (Halibut, Trout, Cod, Flounder, etc.)	1	oz
Tuna; fresh or water packed	1	oz
Clams, Crab, Lobster, Scallops, Shrimp	1	oz
Cheese (≤ 1 gram fat)		
Fat Free Cheese	1	oz
Cheese (≤ 1 gram fat per ounce)	1	oz
Cottage cheese (fat free)	¼	cup
Cottage cheese (2%)	¼	cup
Other		
Egg whites	2	
Egg whites (liquid)	¼	cup
Egg Beaters (liquid)	¼	cup
All Whites (liquid)	4 ½	tbsp

Lean Meats and Meat Substitutes

1 lean meat exchange (0 g CHO, 7 g protein, 3 g fat, 55 calories)

Beef (cooked) USDA Select or Choice grades		
Flank steak	1	oz
Round	1	oz
Sirloin	1	oz
Tenderloin	1	oz
T-Bone steak	1	oz
Pork (cooked)		
Ham	1	oz
Canadian bacon	1	oz
Pork Loin chop	1	oz
Pork tenderloin	1	oz
Lamb (roast, chop, leg)	1	oz
Fish (cooked)		
Catfish	1	oz
Oysters	6	medium
Salmon (fresh or canned)	1	oz
Sardines	2	medium
Tuna (drained oil packed)	1	oz

Continued

Cheese		
Cheese (≤ 1–3 grams fat per ounce)	1	oz
Soy cheese	1.5	slices
Cottage cheese (4.5% fat)	¼	cup
Parmesan Cheese	2	tbsp

Medium Fat Meats and Meat Substitutes

1 medium fat meat exchange (0 g CHO, 7 g protein, 5 g fat, 75 calories)

Beef (cooked)		
Most cuts when trimmed	1	oz
Pork (cooked)		
Pork (top loin, chop, cutlets)	1	oz
Poultry (cooked)		
Chicken/Turkey, dark meat, skin	1	oz
Cheese		
Cheese (≤ 5 grams fat per ounce)	1	oz
Other		
Eggs	1	egg
Soy or Peanut butter (plus 1 fat exchange)	1	tbsp
Tempeh	¼	cup
Tofu (fat & protein content vary by brand; be sure to check label)	4	oz

High Fat Meats and Meat Substitutes

1 medium fat meat exchange (0 g CHO, 7 g protein, 8 g fat, 100 calories)

Cheese (regular)	1	oz
Pork (cooked, spare ribs, barbecue)	1	oz
Sausage (cooked)	1	oz
Soy sausage (cooked)	2	oz
Peanut butter	2	tbsp

Fat Lists

1 fat exchange (0 g CHO, 5 g protein, 5 g fat, 45 calories)

Monounsaturated fats		
5 oz wine 1 Fruit + 1 Fat exchange	1	
Almond butter	½	tbsp
Almonds	6	nuts
Avocado, 4" across	⅛	
Guacamole	2	tbsp
Cashews	6	nuts
Mixed nuts (50% peanuts)	6	nuts
Oil (canola, olive)	1	tsp
Olives, ripe (black)	8	large
Olives, green, stuffed	10	large
Peanut butter	2	tsp
Peanuts	10	nuts
Pecans	4	halves
Pesto sauce	2	tsp
Sesame seeds	1	tbsp
Soy or Peanut butter	1	tbsp
Walnut halves	5	
Polyunsaturated fats		
Brummel & Brown Spread	1	tbsp
Margarine (all forms)	1	tsp
Mayonnaise, reduced fat	1	tbsp
Mayonnaise, regular	1	tsp
Oil (corn, safflower, soybean)	1	tsp
Miracle Whip Salad Dressing; regular	2	tsp
Miracle Whip Salad Dressing; reduced fat	1	tbsp
Saturated fats		
Bacon	1	slice
Butter	1	tsp
Cream (light, coffee, sour)	1	tbsp
Half & half	3	tbsp
Vegetable shortening	1	tsp

Exchange lists adapted with permission from What Works Nutrition Software®

A Final Word on Portion Control

When things are going well, you may wonder why it's necessary to be so exact in tracking your intake. True, my motto is if something's working, don't mess with it! But if you find yourself flagging on the mat or lugging around some extra pounds of dead weight, then it's harder to alter what you're doing if you don't really know what you'd been doing prior. It's impossible to alter a plan if you never knew what that plan was in the first place. To make progress in your martial arts performance and to improve your body composition, you'll have to adopt a scientific approach, which requires consistent, reliable, quantifiable methods to yield quantifiable results.

CHAPTER 10

Rules for Feeding the Machine

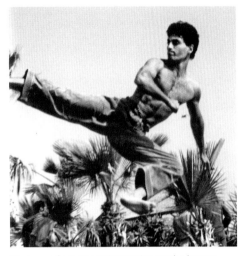

Timing and macronutrient ratios are the keys to building muscle and staying lean.

I hear a lot of fighters who are not as lean as they'd like to be immediately blame their metabolism. I've also had fighter clients who ate only three times a day whine about their energy levels. They blame their genetics or their age, throw up their hands, and say, "When I hit 30 it was all downhill from there." I also have a lot of retired athletes—NFL players to track and field Olympians—who didn't know how to adjust their caloric intake once they'd stopped training at such high volumes. They immediately blamed their metabolism, but after adjusting their eating schedules, determining proper amounts, and tweaking ratios, they were able to get those metabolic engines revving again. There was *nothing* wrong with their resting metabolic rates.

In almost *all* cases, we were able to design plans that would rev up their metabolism. You are the *creator*, not the victim, of your metabolism. With a little science, you can reach your goals regardless of your age or genetics.

In my practice, there are two rules that *all* of my clients must follow. From my bodybuilders who are 4% body fat, to my hard gainers, to my elite athletes, to my clients who are trying to lose body fat—they all start with the same two rules, and then we customize from there. It doesn't matter who you are, these rules have to do with controlling blood sugars and keeping your metabolic fire stoked. They are the foundation of your plan.

Timing Is Everything...
Rule Number One: Eat Every 3 to 4 Hours

I'm sure you've heard this one before: if you go too long without eating, you starve your body and slow your metabolism. Your body is very smart. If you go more than 4 hours without eating your body switches over to survival mode. In an attempt to conserve energy, it slows your metabolism to save energy.

A couple of other things happen in survival mode. Your brain runs on only one kind of fuel—glucose. The problem is your body is only able to store limited amounts of glucose. Within 3 or 4 hours of eating, you're out of blood glucose. Your liver will dump out some reserves, but after that, how do you stay alive? You actually cannibalize your lean muscle tissue and convert it to sugar through a process called gluconeogenesis.

So in that 5th, 6th, 7th hour without eating, you're actually chomping on your own muscle mass to stay alive. Muscle is metabolically active tissue, meaning that it burns calories. Fat does not. So from a composition perspective, you want to keep that muscle around. From an athletic perspective, you may not want to lose muscle because it is integral to speed and power—unlike fat, which is dead weight.

The worst part about eating too infrequently, though, is that even if you make healthy choices—that chicken salad, those egg whites, that whole grain bread—by the time you finally do get to food, most of it gets stored as fat. You'll cause an insulin spike, which we'll discuss below, that causes you to store excess glucose as fat. And because your blood sugars will be so low, you'll be prone to eat much more than you should, and again, excess calories are stored as body fat.

Eating too infrequently is one of the most common problems I see in my practice. Clients will often come in for the first time and tell me they're working out on an empty stomach. If they're taking spin class, I tell them they're literally spinning their wheels. They're tearing down muscle as they think they're building it. They're setting themselves up to *store* body fat as they think they're burning it.

Rule Number Two: Eat Protein with Every Meal and Snack

Rule Number Two has to do with blood sugar control and states that you will never eat carbohydrates by themselves. You will *always* eat protein at every snack and meal.

The reason for this is that carbohydrates are the only nutrients that cause your blood sugars to spike significantly. Normal blood sugars are approximately between 80 and 120 mg/dl. Go below 80, and you're in the basement. If you're like me, you're tired, hungry, dizzy, and cranky. This is also when you start dipping into your muscle tissue as an alternative form of sugar. Go above 120, and your body must secrete a hormone called insulin.

When you eat, your blood glucose rises. This stimulates the pancreas to secrete insulin, which in turn, stimulates the uptake of glucose into cells for use or in its storage form as glycogen. Glycogen is stored in your liver and muscles. When you eat too much, insulin also instigates the storage of excess glucose as fat. Insulin is also the strongest inhibitor of lipolysis (the breakdown of fat) so if leaning out is your goal, keeping insulin levels under control is key.

Conversely, the hormone glucagon is secreted when energy is needed, as it is with exercise, or when insulin levels are low. Glucagon's job is to break down glycogen so that it can be released into the blood as glucose.

As we just said, carbs are the only things that cause your blood sugars to spike. They also do this very quickly. If you eat any carbohydrate by itself—whether that be potatoes, bread, fruit, or refined sugar—it empties out of your stomach very quickly within 20 to 40 minutes. BAM! Out of your stomach, into your bloodstream. This causes a surge in blood sugar. It is this sudden spike in blood sugars that causes a correspondingly swift surge in insulin secretion. Unfortunately, the response is not always perfect and often overshoots the mark, causing a subsequent blood sugar plunge. With your blood sugars in the basement again, guess what you crave? Sugar! If you act on that craving, you'll repeat the pattern of sugar spike, insulin surge, and low blood glucose. This is what we call the sugar high and crash. It occurs whenever the body must handle a sudden and significant glycemic load.

To prevent this cycle from occurring, we turn to protein, which empties out of your stomach much slower than carbs—2 to 3 hours, as opposed to 20 to 40 minutes. When you eat protein with carbs, those carbs have to hang out with the protein. They empty out at the same rate—2 to 3 hours. As a result, you have a much slower, steadier release of sugar into your bloodstream, you stay within the optimal range, and from the time you eat something to the time you're tired, hungry, dizzy, and cranky again is 3 to 4 hours as opposed to 20 to 40 minutes.

In case you're wondering, you should be able to go 3 to 4 hours instead of 2 to 3 hours, because most meals contain a small amount of fat—usually in the protein. Fat has the slowest gastric emptying time—3–5 hours—so it will increase the time you can go between meals.

Not All Carbs Are Created Equal...
Corollary to Rule Number Two: Avoid Concentrated Sugars

The ratios of macronutrients play a huge part in controlling your blood sugars, but the types of carbohydrates you eat are also important. Remember our glycemic index? The corollary to Rule Number Two is similar to the idea of the glycemic index. You want to choose starchy, complex carbs instead of high-glycemic-index, simple sugar carbs.

If you have the food label for a food item, use it. For example, a box of Frosted Flakes has 29 g of total carbohydrates, 12 of those are from sugar. That's 41% sugar. Bye bye, Frosted Flakes. Special K, on the other hand, has 16 g total carbs and 3 grams of sugar. That's 19% sugar. Hello, Special K.

Once again, our goal is to prevent insulin spikes that will promote overeating, fat storage, and sugar cravings. By keeping your blood sugars under control, you promote the release of glucagon, and subsequently the release of fat from storage.

Another benefit to choosing complex and lean proteins for fuel is that your body must *expend* energy to digest that food. This is what we call the thermic effectof food. Protein and complex carbohydrates take more time and energy to break down and assimilate. As we've just learned, part of the advantage is that your blood sugar and, thus, insulin levels won't spike. The other advantage is that the breakdown of protein and complex carbs actually requires you to burn energy as well.

From my work with diabetics who have to monitor their blood sugars daily, I've seen these rules work time and time again. It's not miraculous. It's not rocket science, but it is science. For my athletes, I've seen these rules prevent fatigue and muscle loss while enhancing performance levels.

Later in this book we'll take a look at a few case studies and how following these rules—and not following them—affected progress.

CHAPTER 11

Train Smarter, Not Harder

So far, we've covered all the nutrition variables, but if we really want to reach our fitness goals, we need to look at the other half of the equation. We need to tailor your exercise program so that it works with your eating plan. Otherwise, you might see some results, but it's likely you won't progress past that. The more variables you cover, and the more precisely you cover them, the more efficiently you'll reach your goals.

A VO_2 max test is a great tool for improving your aerobic capacity.

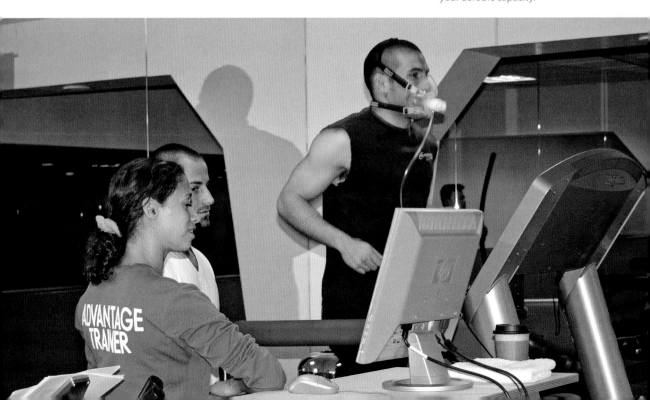

VO$_2$ Max: "Real World Power"

The ability to fight 12 rounds, issue kicking combinations, the ability to *endure* is what is often referred to as "real world power." In physiology terms, this is called cardiorespiratory endurance, which is your body's ability to sustain prolonged exercise. Our measure of cardiorespiratory endurance is a test we call VO$_2$ max. This number tells us the maximal amount of oxygen consumption that can be used to sustain exercise. In short, it is a measurement of aerobic capacity.

Genetics are instrumental in determining your VO$_2$ max, contributing up to 25–50% of variance among individuals. Elite male endurance athletes may have a VO$_2$ max over 90 ml/kg/minute, and elite women athletes may test out at over 70 ml/kg/minute. While genetics are a huge factor, you can still improve your VO$_2$ max with training.

Enter the Heart Rate Monitor

To maximize your genetic potential, you'll want to get a heart rate monitor, which is, in my opinion, one of the most valuable training tools at your disposal. While heart rate itself does not measure VO$_2$ max, it is directly related to oxygen use during exercise. As your heart rate increases, so does your consumption of oxygen as it is delivered to your exercising muscles. As your fitness improves, you may see your heart rate decrease by as much as 10 to 15 beats per minute. This is because your heart has become stronger and is, therefore, able to pump out more blood to your muscles with each beat. You are able to do more work at a lower heart rate. This is why highly conditioned athletes have such low resting pulses. The monitor allows you to track these numbers easily.

By using a monitor, you also aren't chained to a machine to monitor calories or heart rate. You can measure these variables anywhere—in the ring, in the pool, on the beach, in the street, on the side of a mountain.

At the very least, a good monitor should track per session your total calories burned, average heart rate, maximum heart rate, total time, and time spent in your fat-burning zone. Two monitors I recommend are the Polar F6 and F11, which record all of these parameters and store the information for your last 12 workouts. Some monitors also allow you to uplink the information to the web for analysis and permanent data storage.

Determining Exercise Zones

The general formula for determining heart rate zones is to take a percentage from your maximum heart rate. To determine your maximum heart rate, subtract your age from 220:

MHR = 220 – age

Then depending on your goals, you would multiply by the following percentages:

1. 50–60% for rest and recovery
2. 60–70% for fat burning
3. 70–85% for fat burning and aerobic improvement
4. 85–100% for improved aerobic and anaerobic metabolism

So if we had a 33-year-old martial artist looking to improve his ability to withstand anaerobic lactic acid buildup, he would subtract his age from 220:

220 – 33 = 187

His maximum heart rate is 187, which we multiply by 85 and 100 percent, yielding a workout heart rate range between 159 and 187.

VO$_2$ Max Testing

The problem with using the 220-minus-age formula is that there is at least a plus-or-minus-15-beat variance among individuals. I know plenty of men and women clients who can operate at *well over* their estimated maximum heart rate. If they were to train according to this formula, they may not be working hard enough.

Also, if you've been training for awhile, your zones will have shifted over time. You probably have "outgrown" the formula and are able to operate at a much higher intensity. So if you really want to be precise in your training approach, I would suggest doing a VO$_2$ max test or active metabolic assessment.

Implications for Body Composition

Below you'll find a printout from my own VO$_2$ max test in 2005. I show these print-outs to my clients all the time to demonstrate the importance of getting a meta-bolic assessment and monitoring their exercise with a heart rate monitor. The curve shows how many calories I'm burning from fat. Between the heart rates of 124 and 157 beats per minute (BPM), I'm burning the most calories from fat—only 9.9 total calories and 5.4 are coming from fat.

VO$_2$ max test done in 2005

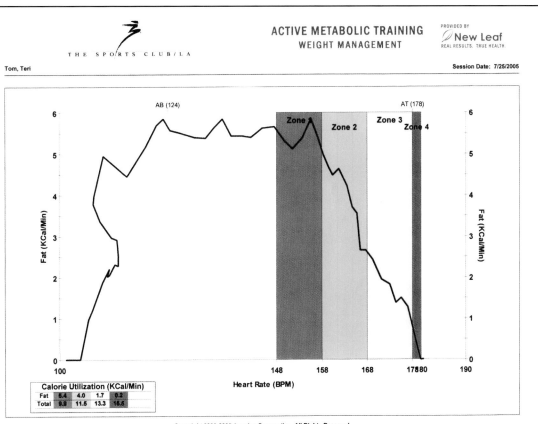

Image courtesy of New Leaf Health and Fitness (www.newleaffitness.com)

As I work harder, you'll see that I'm burning more total calories, but less are com-ing from fat. After 157 BPM, I am still burning fat but am starting to convert some muscle to energy as well. From 158 to 168 BPM, I'm burning 11.5 total calories but only 4 are coming from fat. From 168 to 178 BPM, 13.3 total calories and only 1.7

are from fat. And between 178 and 180 BPM, which is me essentially running up a hill, I'm expending the most calories at 15.5 but almost *none* are coming from fat.

At this point, I am at what we call anaerobic threshold (AT). I am no longer efficiently burning fat. All of my energy is coming from sugars or muscle that is being converted to sugar. As you can imagine, then, it's very important to know where AT occurs and where that fat-burning Zone 1 is.

If I am a martial artist, I certainly don't want to be sacrificing lean tissue. I need to condition my body so that it becomes used to operating at higher levels of intensity without chomping on my muscle.

Likewise, if I am someone who is trying to lean out, it makes no sense for me to exercise at such a high intensity that few of the calories I'm burning are coming from fat. I see this all the time in the gym, especially in group exercise classes, where my clients tend to get so caught up in the loud music and the competitive vibe, they spin their hearts out and cannibalize their lean tissue. One of my clients dropped 4 pounds of muscle the week he started spinning! He was literally spinning his wheels. I made him wear a heart rate monitor after that.

Trainers have a saying—train smarter, not harder. It's counter-intuitive, but exercising harder is not always the right answer, especially if composition is your goal. The same goes for eating. Taking away calories is not always the answer to getting leaner. I can't tell you how many clients have only one blip on their charts indicating a gain in fat and a loss in muscle, and when I ask them what happened that week, they tell me they exercised harder and ate less! Again, in both exercise and nutrition, we're striving to find the right balance between too much and too little. A metabolic assessment and a heart rate monitor can help you find that balance.

Implications for Peak Performance

Not everyone, of course, is trying to lose body fat. For athletes who are looking to improve their performance, a metabolic assessment and heart rate monitor can be great tools. For example, in the ring, you want to be able to fight aerobically at a very high intensity. You want to be able to utilize oxygen and fat over a wider range of heart rate ranges.

With training, the body adapts by increasing stroke volume—your heart is able to pump more blood to your exercising muscles with each beat. Your body also responds metabolically, as we mentioned, by increasing the amount of fat, as opposed to carbohydrate, that you burn, thus sparing lean tissue. At the same time, it also becomes more efficient at keeping down lactate levels within the muscle. This enables you to work at a much higher heart rate while still enabling you to use oxygen and fat to fuel your muscles.

VO$_2$ max test done in 2007

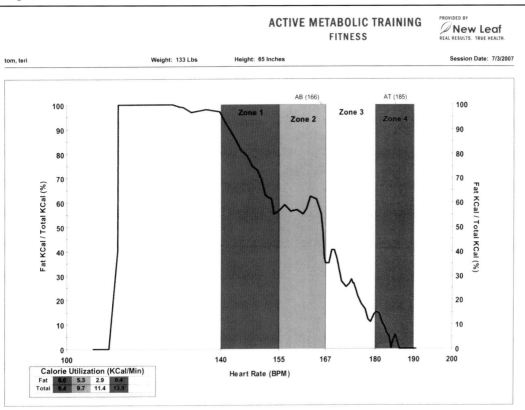

Image courtesy of New Leaf Health and Fitness (www.newleaffitness.com)

To demonstrate some of these adaptations, I've included a VO$_2$ max test I took two years later in 2007 (above). There are several differences between this chart and my test in 2005:

1. **Getting fat-burning systems up and running**. In the 2005 test, you'll see that it takes me a few minutes to reach my peak fat-burning zone. Before my heart rate reaches 124 BPM, there is a gradual increase in fat utilization. Between 0

and 124 BPM, my exercise is being fueled by both the glycolytic and aerobic (oxidative) systems. In 2007, though, notice I go straight into peak fat utilization immediately. Almost from the moment I start, I'm in aerobic mode.

2. **Efficiency of fat utilization and sparing of lean tissue.** From the 2007 test results, notice that within each heart rate zone, in the second test, I am burning fewer total calories but more of those calories are coming from fat than they did in the first test. For instance, in the 125–155 range, in 2005 I burned 9.9 total calories and 5.4 of those were from fat. But in 2007, I burned 8.4 total calories in that same zone, and 6.0 came from fat. A similar pattern is found across all of the zones. What does this mean? I'm burning less total calories, so I'm not burning nearly as many sugars, so there is less need to convert muscle to carbohydrate. My body is better conditioned so I'm able to use much more of my calories from fat via the oxidative system.

3. **Increased aerobic base.** From the 2007 test results, you can also see that I am now able to burn fat—and more of it—over a wider range of heart rate zones. I'm able to get fat-burning systems running faster—almost immediately as opposed to at 125 BPM. In 2007, I'm also burning more calories from fat across all heart rate zones. And I'm able to eke out that last bit of effort at 191 BPM instead of sputtering out at 180. My body is now more efficient at keeping lactate levels down by using oxygen, and I feel that lactic burn much later.

4. **Recovery of fat utilization during test.** Notice in the 2005 test, at about 160, my fat utilization made a small attempt at recovery. This also occurred at around 166 and 176 BPM. Other than those three sites, it was pretty much a steady downward trend toward Anaerobic City. In the 2007 test, notice how those little peaks are more pronounced and more frequent at around 156, 163, 168, 170, 180, and 185 BPM. As the test administrator increased the speed of the treadmill, I dipped further into anaerobic mode. But you'll notice in the 2007 test, once my body adjusted to the increased intensity, it would bounce back and start to use more calories from fat. Of course, the administrator continued to increase the intensity every minute, and after a brief aerobic comeback, the treadmill speed would go up, and I'd continue my descent toward anaerobic threshold.

5. **Greater workload, decreased heart rate.** There's a steep hill that I like to run for interval training. When I first started running it, I couldn't finish without walking part of it. Then I could run it continuously and finish it in 5:30 with my heart rate in the low-to-mid-80s. Now I can finish it in 3:59 at the same heart rate. This is one of the adaptations of interval training. You're able to do more work with each heartbeat.

6. **VO_2 max.** My VO_2 max for this test ended up being 53.6 ml/min. This means I consumed 53.6 milliliters of oxygen per minute for every kilogram of my body weight. Not too shabby for my age group, but considering the highest recorded VO_2 max for a woman is somewhere around 70 ml/min, I've got a way to go. Unfortunately, as we already stated, VO_2 max is determined to a large extent by genetics, age, and sex.

To accomplish these adaptations, we incorporate interval training by alternating between the zones. After my first test, I was told to do intervals between Zones 1 and 4. I might cruise for a few minutes in Zone 1 and then give an all-out effort in Zone 4 for a minute. Then I would back down to Zone 1 again and repeat the process. By getting used to exercising between 170 and 180 BPM, I was able to increase the amount of fat I was burning at those heart rates from 1.7 kcal/min in the first assessment to 2.9 kcal/min in the second.

It may seem like splitting hairs, but when you square off with someone in the ring, you'll notice the difference!

CHAPTER 12

Four Scenarios

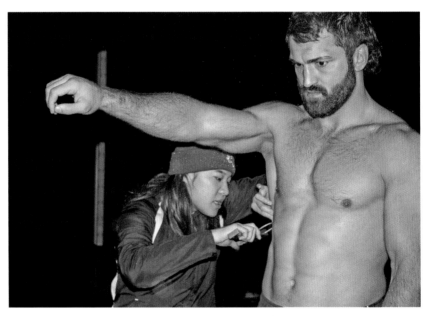

As my clients know all too well, the calipers don't lie. Midaxilla measurement
on Andrei Arlovski. *(Photo: Ariza)*

Now that you know your approximate caloric needs, exercise guidelines, and how
to use the exchange system, have your body fat measured. Then follow one of the
meal plans for one week. Re-measure your body fat. Your results should follow one
of four scenarios. If you've done everything correctly, one of them will give us the
key to what you need to do next. This information is what makes the plan bullet-
proof. If something's not working, you'll know why and simply change it. Here are
the scenarios you will encounter from week to week.

1. **Gaining fat/gaining muscle.** Unless you are trying to put on body fat (and I do have some clients who actually want this), this means your calories are too high. Take them down the next week.

2. **Losing fat/losing muscle.** If you're following the plan to the letter, and unless you are trying to shed muscle, you'll need to increase your protein. Try doing so by a few protein exchanges at a time—maybe by 2 or 3 at lunch and dinner. If you're still losing muscle, increase protein at snacks as well. Doing too much cardio at too high of an intensity would also cause muscle loss, so continue to monitor your workouts.

3. **Losing muscle/gaining fat.** This is often caused by not eating on time. If you wait too long between meals—more than 4 hours—your body goes into starvation mode and slows your metabolism. When you finally get to food, a greater percentage of it is stored as body fat. But assuming you are following the plan and eating on time, this result simply means you aren't getting enough food. You're cannibalizing your muscle tissue and stockpiling the food you do take in as fat. Try increasing calories by increments of 250 to 500 kcal.

4. **Losing fat/gaining muscle.** In most cases, this is exactly what we want. No need to fix what ain't broke. Maintain current plan for as long as it yields these results. If the client wants to lose body fat but not gain muscle, then we would lower the protein intake.

Looking at these scenarios, you can see why I prefer to measure progress based on composition, not weight. Composition gives me so much more information than weight alone. Changes take place by the millimeter. This is usually too gradual for you to notice what's happening. And as I mentioned earlier, most of my de-conditioned clients will *gain* weight the first week. As they build muscle and store more glycogen and water, they may actually weigh more as they're losing body fat.

Imagine how we might panic in the first few weeks, then, if all we had to go on was the client's weight? We'd abandon our fitness plans immediately, which is usually what happens when people try to do this on their own or without the benefit of composition measurements. And imagine trying to make weight for a fight or competition without this information! You wouldn't know whether you were losing fat or muscle, but the difference would be huge in terms of your performance.

By the time clients come to me, they've usually tried every diet, meal plan, and delivery service known to man. Barring rare hormonal imbalances or other conditions that require medical attention (eg thyroid issues, testosterone imbalances, etc) we really can't miss if we cover all the variables. By monitoring a client's body composition, I know whether I need to turn left or right whenever we hit a bump in the road or a plateau. And if we monitor closely, the client will get there sooner. For example, if a client is losing muscle and gaining fat, if he comes in weekly for composition assessment, I'll catch it immediately and make adjustments. He won't go for weeks or months heading in the wrong direction, and we won't have to spend extra time undoing something that could've been taken care of much earlier.

From our discussion on cardiovascular training, also keep in mind that training variables need to be in place as well. This is why the heart rate monitor is so important. I ask my clients to bring their heart rate monitors in every week so I can see what's been happening on the exercise front. If, for example, a client loses muscle on me and I see his average heart rate for most workouts is in the 180s, it's probably not his nutrition plan that is the culprit. It's more likely that he's working too hard and spending too much time exercising anaerobically. Or if I see he's not losing any body fat and his average heart rate is only 110, then he probably needs to step it up.

Always remember the two—exercise and nutrition—work hand in hand.

CHAPTER 13

The Micronutrients

To reach body composition and/or performance goals, we've emphasized manipulation of the macronutrients—carbs, protein, fat. It's important not to forget that the micronutrients—vitamins and minerals—are required for efficient utilization of those macronutrients. Unlike macronutrients, which are consumed in large amounts and are measured in grams, the micronutrients are only required in small amounts and are measured in milligrams and micrograms.

One of the biggest misconceptions about the micronutrients is that they provide energy. Technically, they do not. Vitamins and minerals do not actually provide calories. They are, however, vital in helping our bodies convert the macronutrients into fuel that we can use. So while they themselves do not provide energy, the micronutrients enable us to access the energy stored in macronutrients. On the other hand, intake of only vitamins and minerals would be like trying to run your car with spark plugs but without gasoline. Would you race a car without spark plugs? That's like trying to knife fight without the micronutrients.

In addition to energy metabolism, vitamins and minerals are also essential to structural building, maintenance, and repair. I could, of course, write a book on the micronutrients alone, but for the purposes of this book, I really just want you to know what they do. By knowing the roles that vitamins and minerals play, you'll know why it's important to eat nutrient-dense *real* foods. This is what I call getting the most bang for your buck. Yes, that bleached piece of white bread might give you the same number of calories as a whole-grain bread, but the whole-grain bread is going to give you added vitamins and minerals that have been washed out of the

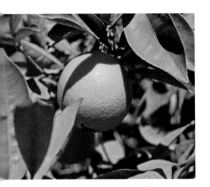

Oranges are packed with micro-nutrients like potassium and vitamin C.

white bread. After reading this chapter, you'll know *why* you benefit from choosing certain vitamin and mineral-rich foods.

And at the end of this chapter, I'll also give my two cents on the controversy of supplementation.

Alphabet Soup: About the Tables

When it comes to nutrient recommendations, there's quite a lot of confusion regarding the DRIs, RDAs, and AIs. RDA stands for "Recommended Dietary Allowance." These were first established in 1941 by the Food and Nutrition Board and were updated every 10 years. The RDAs provide the average dietary intake that prevents a deficiency in 98% of a specified population. Different recommendations are set for different populations (i.e., age groups). The RDAs were developed to determine the *minimum* amounts of nutrients to prevent disease. They were never intended to determine quality of an individual's diet.

In 1997, the Food and Nutrition Board of the National Academy of Sciences revised the RDAs and created the Dietary Reference Intakes (DRI), which included four reference values:

Estimated Average Requirement (EAR): This is the amount of a specific nutrient estimated to meet the needs of 50% of the population and is used for evaluating diets of populations.

Recommended Dietary Allowances (RDA): The average dietary intake that prevents deficiency in 98% of a population.

Adequate Intake (AI): This is an intake goal for a nutrient that does not have a set RDA. Either lack of data, or uncertainty of existing data, do not allow determination with confidence the percentage of individuals covered by this intake.

Tolerable Upper Intake Level (UL): The highest level of nutrient intake that does not produce risk of adverse health effects in 98% of the population. An Upper Intake Level designated ND means that it is not determinable because there is not enough data on the adverse effects of excessive amounts of a nutrient.

In the following charts, if the volumes are in bold type, this is the RDA for that nutrient. If the volume is in ordinary type followed by an asterisk (*), this is an AI value and does not have an established RDA.

Vitamins

Vitamins are organic (carbon-containing) substances that can be divided into the categories water soluble and fat soluble. The water solubles are not stored in large amounts in the body and must be ingested frequently. They include vitamin B1 (thiamin), vitamin B2 (riboflavin), vitamin B6 (pyroxidine), vitamin B12 (cyanoco-balamn), niacin (nicotinmide), pantothenic acid, folic acid (folate, folacin), biotin, and vitamin C (ascorbic acid).

The fat solubles are stored in the body's fatty (adipose) tissue so they do not need to be ingested as frequently as the water solubles, and because of this, they can reach toxic levels when taken in excess. The fat soluble vitamins are A, D, E, and K.

Vitamins are responsible for the following functions:

- Act as co-enzymes to facilitate and regulate energy metabolism
- Act as antioxidants to prevent cell damage
- Support visual function
- Support growth and mineralization of bone
- Support blood-clotting mechanisms
- Control tissue synthesis

Tables 7 and 8 summarize the functions and recommended intakes of the water and fat soluble vitamins, respectively.

Minerals

Minerals are inorganic substances that are divided into the major and trace categories. Major minerals are required in larger amounts (> 100 mg/day) and include calcium, phosphorus, potassium, sulfur, sodium, chlorine (choloride), and magnesium. The trace minerals are required in much smaller amounts (<100 mg/day) and include iron, fluorine (fluoride), zinc, copper, selenium, iodine, and chromium.

Table 7. Water Soluble Vitamins Summary

Water Soluble Vitamins	Function	Sources
Vitamin B1 (thiamin)	part of coenzyme TPP in carbohydrate and branch chain amino acid metabolism, supports normal appetite and nerve function	enriched and fortified bread products, pork, liver, legumes, nuts
Vitamin B2 (riboflavin)	part of coenzyme FMN and FAD for energy metabolism, supports normal vision and skin health	dairy products, organ meats, bread products, fortified cereals, leafy green vegetables
Vitamin B3 (niacin, nictotinic acid, niacinamide)	part of coenzymes NAD and NADP for energy metabolism, supports skin health, supports nervous and digestive systems	all protein-containing foods, nuts, dairy, fortified cereals, enriched and whole-grain breads, nuts
Vitamin B5 (pantothenic acid)	part of coenzyme A for fatty acid metabolism	chicken, beef, potatoes, oats, liver, whole grains, tomato products, yeast, egg yolk, broccoli
Vitamin B6 (pyridoxine, pyridoxal, pyridoxamine)	part of coenzyme PLP and PMP for amino acid and fatty acid metabolism, conversion of tryptophan to niacin, niacin, production of red blood cells	leafy green vegetable, meats, fish, poultry, shellfish, legumes, fruits, whole grains
Vitamin B12 (Cobalamin)	part of coenzyme for amino acid synthesis, protein metabolism, reforms folate coenzyme	animal products including shellfish, eggs, dairy
Biotin	part of coenzyme in fat, glycogen, and amino acid synthesis	liver, fruits, meats
Folic Acid (folate, folacin)	part of coenzyme THF and DHF for DNA synthesis, prevention of neural tube defects	green leafy vegetables, fortified grain products, legumes, seeds, liver
Vitamin C (ascorbic acid)	collagen formation, antioxidant, enhances iron absorption, cofactor in reactions involving copper, promotes resistance to infection	citrus fruits, tomatoes, potatoes, brussels sprouts, cauliflower, broccoli, strawberries, cabbage, spinach

RDA/AI (see page 114)	UL (see page 114)	Deficiency Symptoms	Toxicity Symptoms
Males: **1.2 mg/d** Females: **1.1 mg/d**	ND	edema, enlarged heart, abnormal heart rhythm, heart failure, loss of reflexes, mental confusion, paralysis, weakness, wasting, degeneration	
Males: **1.3 mg/d** Females: **1.1 mg/d**	ND	cracks at corners of mouth, inflamed eyeleds, sensitivity to light, reddening of cornea, skin rash	
Males: **16 mg/d** Females: **14 mg/d**	Males: 35 mg/d Females: 35 mg/d	diarrhea, inflamed tongue, loss of appetite, weakness, altered mental status, dermatitis	nausea, vomiting, diarrhea, dizziness, rash, liver damage, low blood pressure
Males: 5 mg/d* Females: 5 mg/d*	ND	vomiting, intestinal distress, insomnia, fatigue	diarrhea, water retention
Males: **1.3 mg/d, 1.7 mg/d** (50-70 yrs), **1.7 mg/d** (>70 yrs) Females: **1.3 mg/d, 1.5 mg/d** (50-70 yrs), **1.5 mg/d** (>70 yrs)	Males: 100 mg/d Females: 100 mg/d	anemia, cracked corners of mouth, irritability, muscle twitching, convulsions, dermatitis, kidney stones, irritation of sweat glands	bloating, depression, fatigue, nerve damage, muscle weakness, bone pain
Males: **2.4 µg/d** Females: **2.4 µg/d**	ND	anemia, fatigue, degeneration of peripheral nerves, paralysis, skin hypersensitivity	
Males: 20 µg/d* Females: 30 µg/d*	ND	loss of appetite, nausea, depression, muscle pain, weakness, fatigue, dermatitis, hair loss	
Males: **400 µg/d** Females: **400 µg/d**	Males: 1,000 µg/d Females: 1,000 µg/d	anemia, diarrhea, constipation, frequent infections, depression, fatigue	masks vitamin B12 deficiency
Males: **90 mg/d** Females: **75 mg/d**	Males: 2,000 mg/d Females: 2,000 mg/d	anemia, pinpoint hemorrhages, frequent infections, bleeding gums, loosened teeth, muscle degeneration and pain, bone fragility, joint pain, rough skin, poor wound healing	nausea, abdominal cramps, diarrhea, headache, fatigue, insomnia, hot flashes, rashes, aggravation of gout symptoms, kidney stones

Volumes shown in **bold**: RDA for that nutrient.
Volumes shown in non-bold with (*): AI value; no established RDA.

Table 8. Fat Soluble Vitamins Summary

Fat Soluble Vitamins	Function	Sources	RDA/AI (see page 114)
Vitamin A (retinol, beta-carotene, carotenoids)	vision, maintenance of epithelial cells, mucous membranes, skin, immune function, reproduction, bone and teeth growth	enriched and fortified bread products, pork, liver, legumes, nuts, eggs, butter, fortified butter substitutes, dark green leafy vegetables, deep orange fruits and vegetables	Males: **900 μg/d** Females: **700 μg/d**
Vitamin D (calciferol, cholecalciferol)	mineralization (building) of bones, regulation of serum calcium and phosphorus concentrations	fortified dairy products, fortified butter substitutes, egg yolks, liver, fatty fish	Males: 5 μg/d*, 10 μg/d (50-70 yrs)*, 15 μg/d (>70 yrs)* Females: 5μg/d*, 10 μg/d (50-70 yrs)*, 15 μg/d (>70 yrs)*
Vitamin E (alpha-tocopherol, tocopherol, tocotrienol)	antioxidant, maintenance of cell membranes and red blood cells, antioxidant protection of Vitamin A and polyunsaturated fatty acids	plant oils, green leafy vegetables, wheat germ, egg yolks, whole grains, nuts, seeds, liver	Males: **15 mg/d** Females: **15 mg/d**
Vitamin K (menadione, phylloquinone)	promotes blood clotting, coenzyme for protein synthesis in blood clotting and bone metabolism	synthesized in digestive tract, green leafy vegetables, plant oils, milk	Males: 120 μg/d* Females: 90 μg/d*

Functions of minerals include:

- Provide structure in bones and teeth (these constitute about 4% of our body mass)
- Maintenance of normal heart function, muscular contraction, neural activity, and acid/base balance
- Regulation of cellular metabolism by becoming parts of enzymes and hormones

UL (see page 114)	Deficiency Symptoms	Toxicity Symptoms
Males: 3,000 µg/d Females: 3,000 µg/d	cessation of bone growth, painful joints, dental decay, anemia, night blindness, gray spots on eye, irreversible drying of eyes, blindness (corneal degeneration), plugging of hair follicles (hyperkeratosis), immune suppression, kidney stones	decalcification, joint pain, stunted growth, pressure inside skull, headaches, loss of hemoglobin and potassium, cessation of menstruation, slowed blood clotting, skin dryness, rash, bleeding lips, nosebleeds, brittle nails, vomiting, diarrhea, overstimulation of immune response, loss of appetite, muscle weakness, fatigue, irritability, jaundice, liver enlargement, fatty liver
Males: 50 µg/d Females: 50 µg/d	rickets (in children), osteomalacia (deformity of limbs, softening of bones, bone fractures), decreased calcium absorption, increased phosphorous absorption, muscle twitching, muscle spasms, lax muscles	increased calcium withdrawal from bones, loss of appetite, weakness, fatigue, increased calcium excretion, calcification of soft tissues, death
Males: 1,000 mg/d Females: 1,000 mg/d	anemia (due to breakage of red blood cells), muscle degeneration, weakness, leg muscle pain	enhances anti-clotting medication effects
ND	hemorrhaging	interferes with anti-clotting medications, brain damage, red blood cell hemolysis

Volumes shown in **bold**: RDA for that nutrient.
Volumes shown in non-bold with (*): AI value; no established RDA.

- Function as electrolytes (sodium, potassium, and chlorine), which modulate fluid exchange within the body's various compartments

Tables 9 and 10 summarize the recommended intakes and functions of the major and trace minerals, respectively.

Table 9. Major Minerals Summary

Major Minerals	Function	Sources
Sodium	electrolyte, maintains fluid and electrolyte balance, nerve impulse transmission, muscle contraction	table salt, soy sauce, pickled foods, processed foods, bread products, meat, canned soups
Chloride	electrolyte, maintans fluid and electrolyte balance, part of hydrochloric acid in stomach, digestion	table salt, soy sauce, pickled foods, processed foods, bread products, meat, canned soups
Potassium	electrolyte, maintains fluid and electrolyte balance, facilitates reactions, cell integrity, nerve impulse, muscle contraction	meats, milk, fruits, vegetables, grains, legumes, all whole foods
Calcium	mineral central to bones and teeth, muscle contraction and relaxation, nerve function, blood clotting, blood pressure, immune function	dairy products, small fish (with bones), tofu, dark green vegetables, legumes
Phosphorus	mineral central to bones and teeth, genetic material, part of phospholipids, energy transfer and buffer in acid-base balance	all animal tissues and animal products
Magnesium	bone mineralization, protein synthesis, enzyme action, muscle contraction, nerve transmission, dental health, immune function	nuts, legumes, whole grains, dark green vegetables, seafood, cocoa
Sulfur	formation of disulfide bridged in building of protein, part of vitamins biotin and thiamin, part of insulin	all proteins (both plant and animal)

RDA/AI (see page 114)	UL (see page 114)	Deficiency Symptoms	Toxicity Symptoms
Males: 1.5 g/d*, 1.3 (50-70 yrs)*, 1.2 g/d (>70 yrs)* Females: 1.5 g/d*, 1.3 (50-70 yrs)*, 1.2 g/d (>70 yrs)*	Males: 2.3 g/d Females: 2.3 g/d	muscle cramps, appetite loss, altered mental status	edema, acute hypertension, increased risk of cardiovascular disease and stroke
Males: 2.3 g/d*, 2.0 (50-70 yrs)*, 1.8 g/d (>70 yrs)* Females: 2.3 g/d*, 2.0 (50-70 yrs)*, 1.8 g/d (>70 yrs)*	Males: 3.6 g/d Females: 3.6 g/d	does not occur under normal circumstances	vomiting, hypertension
Males: 4.7 g/d* Females: 4.7 g/d*	No UL	weakness, confusion, paralysis	weakness, vomiting, can stop heart if given intravenously, hyperkalemia and sudden death in those with renal insufficiency
Males: 1,000 mg/d*, 1,200 mg/d (50-70 yrs)*, 1,200 mg/d (>70 yrs)* Females: 1,000 mg/d*, 1,200 mg/d (50-70 yrs)*, 1,200 mg/d (>70 yrs)*	Males: 2,500 mg/d Females: 2,500 mg/d	stunted growth, bone loss	constipation, kidney stones, malabsorption of other minerals
Males: **700 mg/d** Females: **700 mg/d**	Males: 4,000 mg/d, 4,000 mg/d (50-70 yrs), 3,000 mg/d (>70 yrs) Females: 4,000 mg/d, 4,000 mg/d (50-70 yrs), 3,000 mg/d (>70 yrs)	weakness, bone pain, bone loss	low blood calcium
Males: **350 mg/d** Females: **320 mg/d**	Males: 420 mg/d Females: 350 mg/d	weakness, confusion, convulsions, decreased muscle control, difficulty swallowing, hallucinations	diarrhea (supplements only)
	No UL	not known (would have to occur with protein deficiency symptoms as well)	suppression of growth (due to excess of sulfur-containing amino acids)

Volumes shown in **bold**: RDA for that nutrient.
Volumes shown in non-bold with (*): AI value; no established RDA.

Table 10. Trace Minerals Summary

Trace Minerals	Function	Sources	RDA/AI (see page 114)
Iron	part of hemoglobin for oxygen transport, part of myoglobin which provides oxygen for muscle contraction, cell metabolism	red meat, fish, poultry, shellfish, eggs, legumes, dried fruits, fortified cereals	Males: **8 mg/d** Females: **18 mg/d,** **8 mg/d** (50-70 yrs), **8 mg/d** (>70 yrs)
Zinc	part of enzymes, genetic material, immune function, transport of vitamin A, taste perception, wound healing, sperm production, fetus development, protein production	all proteins, meat, fish, poultry, whole grains, vegetables	Males: **11 mg/d** Females: **8 mg/d**
Iodine	part of thyroid hormones that regulate growth and metabolic rate	iodized salt, seafood, bread, dairy, plants grown in iodine-rich soil, animals that eat iodine-rich foods	Males: **150 µg/d** Females: **150 µg/d**
Selenium	works with vitamin E as antioxidant	seafood, meat, grains	Males: **55 µg/d** Females: **55 µg/d**
Copper	absorption of iron (in hemoglobin), part of enzymes	organ meats, nuts, seeds, wheat bran, cereals, whole grains, cocoa, drinking water	Males: **900 µg/d** Females: **900 µg/d**
Manganese	facilitation of enzyme function, bone formation	nuts, legumes, tea, whole grains	Males: **2.3 mg/d** Females: **1.8 mg/d**
Fluoride	bone and teeth formation, resistance to dental decay	fluoridated drinking water, tea, seafood	Males: **4 mg/d** Females: **3 mg/d**
Chromium	maintenance of blood glucose levels	meat, poultry, fish, beer, vegetable oils, some cereals	Males: 35 µg/d*, 30 µg/d (50-70 yrs)*, 30 µg/d (>70 yrs)* Females: 25 µg/d*, 20 µg/d(50-70 yrs)*, 20 µg/d (>70 yrs)*
Molybdenum	cofactor for enzymes for catabolism of sulfur amino acids, purines, pyridines	legumes, cereals, organ meats	Males: **45 µg/d** Females: **45 µg/d**

UL (see page 114)	Deficiency Symptoms	Toxicity Symptoms
Males: 45 mg/d Females: 45 mg/d	blue sclera, compromised immune function, reduced physical fitness, fatigue, reduced mental function, impaired vision, impaired reactivity, pale nailbeds, concave nails, impaired wound healing, itching, palm creases, reduced resistance to cold, inability to regulate body temperature, pica	infections, lethargy, joint disease, pigmentation, hair loss, death by accidental poisoning (children), organ damage, enlarged liver, amenorrhea, impotence
Males: 40 mg/d Females: 40 mg/d	high ammonia, low alkaline phosphatase, low insulin, stunted growth, impaired collagen synthesis, poor taste and smell, weight loss, delayed glucose absorption, diarrhea, impaired folate absorption, night blindness, delayed onset of puberty, impaired thyroid function, impaired adrenocortical hormone synthesis, low white blood cell count, impaired immune function, liver and spleen enlargement, anorexia, irritability, hair loss, dry skin	anemia, high LDL, low HDL, decreased calcium and copper absorption, diarrhea, vomiting, fever, high white blood cell count, renal failure, muscular pain, lack of coordination, degeneration of heart muscle, dizziness, exhaustion, reproductive failure
Males: 1,100 µg/d Females: 1,100 µg/d	simple goiter, cretinism, thyroid enlargement, weight gain	thyroid enlargement, depressed thyroid activity
Males: 400 µg/d Females: 400 µg/d	predisposition to heart disease, fibrous cardiac tissue	digestive system disorders, hair loss, skin lesions, tooth damage, nervous system dysfunction
Males: 10,000 µg/d Females: 10,000 µg/d	anemia	gastrointestinal distress, liver damage
Males: 11 mg/d Females: 11 mg/d	in animal studies, stunted growth, nervous system disorders, reproductive disorders	neurotoxicity
Males: 10 mg/d Females: 10 mg/d	tooth decay	enamel and skin fluorosis (discoloration), GI distress
ND	glucose intolerance	chronic renal failure
Males: 2,000 µg/d Females: 2,000 µg/d	unknown	gout-like symptoms

Volumes shown in **bold**: RDA for that nutrient.
Volumes shown in non-bold with (*): AI value; no established RDA.

Supplements

To supplement or not to supplement. The debate has divided dietitians for decades. Part of the confusion stems from the fact that there is a huge discrepancy between the needs of active and sedentary people. The Recommended Daily Allowances (RDAs) and the Daily Reference Intakes (DRIs) were based on amounts of nutrients needed to avoid deficiency diseases like rickets, scurvy, and pellagra. These are recommendations that will prevent presentation of clinical symptoms. However, this does not mean that the amounts are adequate for protection at the subclinical level. It is now believed that degenerative diseases due to chronic inflammation start at the subclinical level. Indeed, many cancers are only discovered at advanced levels. Diseases and conditions linked to systemic inflammation include allergies, Alzheimer's disease, arthritis, cancer, diabetes, asthma, fibromyalgia, hypertension, heart attack, irritable bowel disorder, renal failure, lupus, osteoporosis, metabolic syndrome, and stroke.

It is very characteristic of Western medicine to treat the problem after something has already broken, but after 20 years of taking an anti-vitamin stance, the American Medical Association has finally turned a 180, as I find more of my clients' doctors are recommending that they take a daily multivitamin.

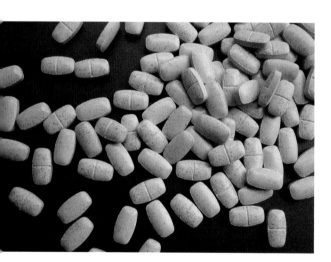

When choosing a supplement, its bioavailability is one important issue to evaluate.

However, because the Food and Drug Administration still does not regulate supplements, there is always the danger of vitamin and mineral toxicity and the question of product quality. As you've seen from the tables in this chapter, the DRIs as determined by the Institute of Medicine (IOM) of the USA National Academy, lists Tolerable Upper Intake Levels (UL). The recommendations in this chapter are for males and females ages 19 to 70. If an "ND" appears under the UL column, then a UL has not yet been determined due to lack of data of adverse effects for excessive intake of that nutrient. For more comprehensive charts that account for infants, children, pregnancy, and lactation, visit www.nal.usda.gov.

Once again, though, keep in mind that the DRIs are the recommendations determined to prevent clinical symptoms and do not take into account the activity level or physiological stresses incurred by an individual. Intense physical exercise places great oxidative stress on the body at the cellular level. And as we've mentioned throughout this book, the martial arts, with their emphasis on impact, demand special care when it comes to recovery methods. Without a sufficient supply of antioxidants, the body is unable to ward off the damage incurred by free radicals generated by stressors like exercise, pollutants, pesticides, etc. And even if your diet is very clean, you are probably still not getting everything you need because of the depletion of nutrients from the soil due to commercial farming processes.

Perhaps an even more important issue than toxicity levels is that of content and purity. For example, lead contamination is a common problem in the production of calcium supplements. Another important quality concern is the supplement's bioavailability. If a supplement does not disintegrate properly, your vitamins and minerals just go out the back door and are not utilized by the body. Poor quality supplements are often excreted in the same pill form as when they were ingested!

So how does one go about finding a supplement that is both safe and effective? For my clients I recommend going to some of the better-known third-party watchdog sites. SupplementWatch.com and ConsumerLab.com are my favorites. In 2007, ConsumerLab published their findings on 39 brands of dietary supplements—an alarming 12 brands failed tests for purity and content. In another ConsumerLab test, less than half of 21 products passed for labeling and quality standards. So even if you think you're getting the proper amounts of nutrients, this really may not be the case due to poor quality products.

My clients, particularly my endurance and professional athletes, have had dramatic improvements in their performance and recovery with these products. And almost all of my clients who have taken quality, pharmaceutical-grade products regularly have reported drastically reduced muscle soreness after workouts.

CHAPTER 14

Ergogenic Aids

I'm a cautious proponent of so-called ergogenic aids and herbal supplements, because according to the FDA website, "The FDA can only take action against products that are not safe or products that make false claims after they are for sale." This means that supplement companies are innocent until proven guilty. This doesn't mean, then, that everything on the market is necessarily safe, let alone beneficial.

That's not to say that all supplements are ineffectual or unsafe. I regularly recommend protein supplements, multi-vitamins and minerals, and some of my clients seem to have had very good results with branch chain amino acids, MCT oil, glucosamine, and glutamine. The problem is that since the FDA doesn't really regulate supplements unless they present a clear health risk, it's hard to pinpoint which ones actually work and meet quality standards.

Even worse, sometimes research is either funded by interested parties to back their own motives. Or existing studies are taken out of context and spun in such a way that falsely supports claims by manufacturers.

Because of this, other than a good multivitamin and mineral, I'm generally uncomfortable rec-

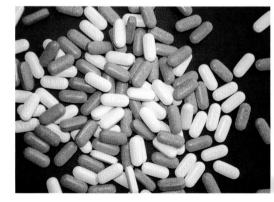

Ergogenic aids can be helpful, but be sure to do your research on specific products and brands before trying them.

ommending specific supplements to clients. What I usually do is arm them with a few reputable sources. They can read the existing research and know who might have funded those studies. From there, they can weigh the information and decide for themselves. The following sites should be helpful in your evaluation of supplements and their manufacturers:

National Council Against Health Fraud
www.ncahf.rg

Quackwatch
www.quackwatch.org

ConsumerLab
www.consumerlab.com

Consumers Union
www.consumersunion.org

Supplement Watch
www.supplementwatch.com

The Hit List

Although I don't recommend supplements to all of my clients, occasionally I do, especially for those who are at the elite or near-elite level. The following are a few of the supplements with which some of my clients have had success. Again, brands, amounts, and need for a particular ergogenic aid vary from individual to individual. Also see the previous chapter on micronutrients for multivitamin and mineral supplement recommendations. Be sure to do your own research, check with your doctor, and evaluate from there.

Omega-3 Fatty Acids

The benefits of the omega-3s are legion, but for athletes, the main benefits are in regards to blood flow and inflammation. Studies have shown that omega-3s may help increase blood flow by up to 36% during exercise. The increased circulation of red blood cells means more efficient transport of oxygen and nutrients through-out the body.

Also of interest to athletes is the reduced inflammation associated with omega-3 intake. Reduced inflammation, of course, means less damage to cells and muscle tissue, resulting in faster post-exercise recovery.[23, 24]

While you can supplement with omega-3 capsules, excessive intake can result in an inability to form blood clots. If you don't want to bleed to death from your next paper cut, check with your doctor before supplementing and limit your omega-3 intake to food sources like fish and flax seed.

Branched-Chain Amino Acids

We've already defined amino acids in the protein chapter. With exercise, the essential amino acids isoleucine, leucine, and valine—collectively, referred to as the branched-chain amino acids (BCAAs)—are gradually depleted with exercise. Studies have shown that supplementation of these amino acids my reduce damage to muscles and, therefore, speed recovery.[25] They may also have a muscle-sparing effect. In clinical settings, BCAAs are sometimes used in cases of severe burns or trauma because of their anticatabolic effect. While BCAAs may not have a direct effect on performance, their roles in recovery and muscle sparing may be beneficial to athletes.[26]

Creatine

Remember from our discussion of the energy systems that the phospho-creatine system powers short bursts of all-out activity. Creatine and phosphorus combine to form phospho-creatine. This allows for the production of ATP, or energy.[27]

By having more creatine circulating in your muscles, you'll be more efficient producing energy. This is useful for eking out that last bit of maximal work output. Creatine is, therefore, best used for anaerobic sports, for both power and endurance. And since boxing and the martial arts have a strong anaerobic component, creatine may be a supplement that would improve performance.[28] If you compete, however, creatine can also cause water retention and may hinder your ability to make weight.

L-Glutamine

Glutamine is the most frequently occurring non-essential amino acid in the human body and is stored in muscle. Under metabolically stressful conditions (i.e., trauma, burns, cancer, sepsis, and infection) it is required in quantities greater than the body can produce and must be taken exogenously. L-glutamine prevents breakdown of muscle tissue, bolsters overall immune function, and protects the mucosal barrier of the intestine. In hospital settings, it is now used in total parenteral nutrition. Glutamine may also increase levels of growth hormone.

The oxidative stress of exercise can deplete skeletal muscle of L-glutamine. Supplementation may, therefore, have muscle sparing and immune-strengthening effects.[29, 30]

Glucosamine and Chondroitin

Studies suggest that glucosamine and chondroitin alleviate the symptoms of osteoarthritis. What isn't known is the mechanism by which this would occur. It seems that glucosamine, an amino monosaccharide, has anti-inflammatory properties and contributes to cartilage repair. It seems to have antioxidant benefits as well. Still, the process by which glucosamine improves symptoms of joint pain is unknown. What is known is that it is a key component of aggrecan, which gives cartilage its shock absorbing qualities.

Similarly, the mechanism by which chondroitin contributes to joint health is also unknown. Like glucosamine, chondroitin is a major component of aggrecan. Studies have suggested that the two work synergistically in improving joint health by slowing the degeneration of cartilage.[31, 32, 33]

CHAPTER 15

Functional Foods

Getting the Most Nutrition Bang for Your Buck

The term "functional food" is something of a buzzword these days. Basically the term describes any food that does more than merely provide energy or the normal spectrum of vitamins and minerals. A functional food may have a specific effect on body processes or have a certain link with a particular disease.

New studies and articles come out every day touting the benefits of certain functional foods. It's beyond the scope of this book to provide a comprehensive list of these, but I'm providing a few examples to make a point—there's no substitute for real food. As you'll see, there are loads of components that have very protective health benefits, and they can't be found in a bar, shake, or pill.

I'm not against the use of meal replacements, protein supplements, or vitamin supplements. But you should try to get in as much "real" food as possible, because there are other nutrients you'll miss out on. Think of your recommended caloric intake as a budget. You only have so many calories to work with. You want to make the most of those calories. You want the most nutrient bang for your caloric buck. With supplements, yes, you get protein, carbs, and fat. And maybe you'll get some vitamins with them. But with real food, you get so much more—fiber, carotenoids, essential fatty acids, flavonoids, plant stanols, probiotics, the list continues to grow. A lot of these functional foods have antioxidant and anti-inflammatory properties, which as we've said repeatedly, are necessary for recovery from exercise, especially the micro and not-so-micro trauma of the martial arts.

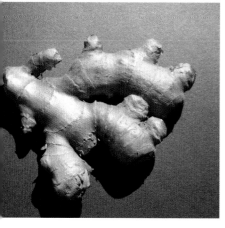

Functional properties of ginger include stimulant, analgesic, sedative, antipyretic, carminative, and antibacterial properties.

Table 11 lists some examples of functional foods and what the components in these foods can do for you. As you'll see, most foods simultaneously fulfill more than a few functions. With all the extra benefits that come with real food, supplements just can't compete.

Table 11. Examples of Functional Food Components

Class/Compound	Sources*	Potential Benefit
Carotenoids		
Beta-carotene	carrots, pumpkin, sweet potato, cantaloupe	neutralizes free radicals, which may damage cells; bolsters cellular antioxidant defenses; can be made into vitamin A in the body
Lutein, Zeaxanthin	kale, collards, spinach, corn, eggs, citrus	may contribute to maintenance of healthy vision
Lycopene	tomatoes and processed tomato products, watermelon, red/pink grapefruit	may contribute to maintenance of prostate health
Dietary (functional and total) Fiber		
Insoluble fiber	wheat bran, corn bran, fruit skins	may contribute to maintenance of a healthy digestive tract; may reduce the risk of some types of cancer
Beta glucan**	oat bran, oatmeal, oat flour, barley, rye	may reduce risk of coronary heart disease (CHD)
Soluble fiber**	psyllium seed husk, peas, beans, apples, citrus fruit	may reduce risk of CHD and some types of cancer
Whole grains**	cereal grains, whole wheat bread, oatmeal, brown rice	may reduce risk of CHD and some types of cancer; may contribute to maintenance of healthy blood glucose levels

* Examples are not an all-inclusive list.
** FDA-approved health claims established for component.

Continued

Table 11 (continued)

Class/Compound	Sources*	Potential Benefit
Fatty Acids		
Monounsaturated fatty acids (MUFAs)**	tree nuts, olive oil, canola oil	may reduce risk of CHD
Polyunsaturated fatty acids (PUFAs) - Omega 3 fatty acids - ALA	walnuts, flax	may contribute to maintenance of heart health; may contribute to maintenance of mental and visual function
PUFAs - Omega 3 fatty acids - DHA/EPA**	salmon, tuna, marine and other fish oils	may reduce risk of CHD; may contribute to maintenance of mental and visual function
Conjugated linoleic acid (CLA)	beef and lamb; some cheese	may contribute to maintenance of desirable body composition and healthy immune function
Flavonoids		
Anthocyanins - Cyanidin, Delphinidin, Malvidin	berries, cherries, red grapes	bolsters cellular antioxidant defenses; may contribute to maintenance of brain function
Flavanols - Catechins, Epicatechins, Epigallocatechin, Procyanidins	tea, cocoa, chocolate, apples, grapes	may contribute to maintenance of heart health
Flavones - Hesperetin, Naringenin	citrus foods	neutralize free radicals, which may damage cells; bolster cellular antioxidant defenses
Flavonols - Quercetin, Kaempferol, Isorhamnetin, Myricetin	onions, apples, tea, broccoli	neutralize free radicals, which may damage cells; bolster celluar antioxidant defenses
Proanthocyanidins	cranberries, cocoa, apples, strawberries, grapes, wine, peanuts, cinnamon	may contribute to maintenance of urinary tract health and heart health
Isothiocyanates		
Sulforaphane	cauliflower, broccoli, brussels sprouts, cabbage, kale, horseradish	may enhance detoxification of undesirable compounds; bolsters cellular antioxidant defenses

* Examples are not an all-inclusive list.
** FDA-approved health claims established for component.

Continued

Table 11 (continued)

Class/Compound	Sources*	Potential Benefit
Minerals		
Calcium**	sardines, spinach, yogurt, low-fat dairy products, fortified foods and beverages	may reduce the risk of osteoporosis
Magnesium**	spinach, pumpkin seeds, whole grain breads and cereals, halibut, brazil nuts	may contribute to maintenance of normal muscle and nerve function, healthy immune function, and bone health
Potassium**	potatoes, low-fat dairy products, whole grain breads and cereals, citrus juices, beans, bananas	may reduce the risk of high blood pressure and stroke, in combination with a low-sodium diet
Selenium	fish, red meat, grains, garlic, liver, eggs	neutralizes free radicals, which may damage cells; may contribute to healthy immune function
Phenolic Acids		
Caffeic acid, Ferulic acid	apples, pears, citrus fruits, some vegetables, coffee	may bolster cellular antioxidant defenses; may contribute to maintenance of healthy vision and heart health
Plant Stanols/Sterols		
Free stanols/Sterols**	corn, soy, wheat, wood oils, fortified foods and beverages	may reduce risk of CHD
Stanol, Sterol esters**	fortified table spreads, stanol ester dietary supplements	may reduce risk of CHD
Polyols		
Sugar alcohols** - Xylitol, Sorbitol, Mannitol, Lactitol	some chewing gums and other food applications	may reduce risk of dental caries
Prebiotics		
Inulin, Fructo-oligosaccharides (FOS), Polydextrose	whole grains, onions, some fruits, garlic honey, leeks, fortified foods and beverages	may improve gastrointestinal health; may improve calcium absorption

* Examples are not an all-inclusive list.
** FDA-approved health claims established for component.

Continued

Table 11 (continued)

Class/Compound	Sources*	Potential Benefit
Probiotics		
Yeast, Lactobacilli, Bifido-bacteria, and other specific strains of beneficial bacteria	certain yogurts and other cultured dairy and non-dairy applications	may improve gastrointestinal health and systemic immunity; benefits are strain-specific
Phytoestrogens		
Isoflavones - Daidzein, Genistin	soybeans and soy-based foods	may contribute to maintenance of bone health, healthy brain and immune function; for women, may contribute to maintenance of menopausal health
Lignans	flax, rye, some vegetables	may contribute to maintenance of heart health and healthy immune function
Soy Protein		
Soy protein**	soybeans and soy-based foods	may reduce risk of CHD
Sulfides/Thiols		
Diallyl sulfide, Allyl methyl trisulfide	garlic, onions, leeks, scallions	may enhance detoxification of undesirable compounds; may contribute to maintenance of heart health and healthy immune function
Dithiolthiones	cruciferous vegetables	may enhance detoxification of undesirable compounds; may contribute to maintenance of healthy immune function
Vitamins		
A***	organ meats, milk, eggs, carrots, sweet potato, spinach	may contribute to maintenance of healthy vision, immune function, and bone health; may contribute to cell integrity
B1 (Thiamin)	lentils, peas, long-grain brown rice, brazil nuts	may contribute to maintenance of mental function; helps regulate metabolism
B2 (Riboflavin)	lean meats, eggs, green leafy vegetables	helps support cell growth; helps regulate metabolism

Continued

Table 11 (continued)

Class/Compound	Sources*	Potential Benefit
B3 (Niacin)	dairy products, poultry, fish, nuts, eggs	helps support cell growth; helps regulate metabolism
B5 (Pantothenic acid)	organ meats, lobster, soybeans, lentils	helps regulate metabolism and hormone synthesis
B6 (Pyroxidine)	beans, nuts, legumes, fish, meat, whole grains	may contribute to maintenance of healthy immune function; helps regulate metabolism
B9 (Folate)**	beans, legumes, citrus foods, green leafy vegetables, fortified breads and cereals	may reduce a woman's risk of having a child with a brain or spinal cord defect
B12 (Cobalamin)	eggs, meat, poulty, milk	may contribute to maintenance of mental function; helps regulate metabolism and supports blood cell formation
Biotin	liver, salmon, dairy, eggs, oysters	helps regulate metabolism and hormone synthesis
C	guava, sweet red/green pepper, kiwi, citrus fruit, strawberries	neutralizes free radicals, which may damage cells; may contribute to maintenance of bone health and immune function
D	sunlight, fish, fortified foods and beverages such as milk, juices, and cereals	helps regulate calcium and phosphorous; helps contribute to bone health; may contribute to healthy immune function; helps support cell growth
E	sunflower seeds, almonds, hazelnuts, turnip greens	neutralizes free radicals, which may damage cells; may contribute to healthy immune function and maintenance of heart health

Adapted with permission from the International Food Information Council Foundation (IFIC)

* Examples are not an all-inclusive list.
** FDA-approved health claims established for component.
*** Preformed vitamin A is found in foods that come from animals. Provitamin A carotenoids are found in many darkly colored fruits and vegetables and are a major source of vitamin A for vegetarians.

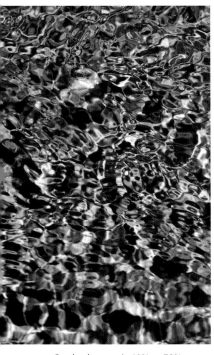

Our body mass is 40% to 70% water.

CHAPTER 16

Fluids: "Be Water My Friend"

Bruce Lee was actually right. We *are* water. In fact, 40 to 70% of our body mass consists of water. Water accounts for 65–75% of muscle weight, 30% of bones, and 93% of blood. You've probably heard that we can go for quite some time without food, but without water, we are toast within days.

Makes sense given that water is the medium in which so many of our bodily functions occur. Nutrients are delivered and metabolic waste products are removed via water. Digestion and absorption of nutrients require water. In respiration, gases are exchanged through water. Life-sustaining chemical reactions occur in water.

Water is present in cells, outside cells, and between cells. It is necessary in the formation of protein and glycogen molecules. From a structural standpoint, it provides turgor for body tissues, giving them form.

Two functions of water should be of particular interest to athletes and martial artists—as a major component of your cooling system and as protection for various parts of your body, most important of which, is yer noggin.

Cooling System

First, water is your body's main cooling system. Your body likes to maintain a temperature somewhere around 98.6°F. Very small deviations from this preferred core temperature result in significant reductions in performance and very unpleasant symptoms. Only 11.5°F more than this and you will literally cook to death. When you exercise, you generate up to an additional 20 times more heat. So why don't we fry to death during exercise? Two reasons. One, during exercise, blood moves closer to the skin to allow heat to radiate away from the body. The second way we cool ourselves is by sweating, which enables us to evaporate heat away from the body via the skin.

Water as Protection

The second role of water, which should be considered important to athletes in contact sports, is water's place as the major constituent of so many bodily fluids. These include the synovial fluid that lubricates your joints and the cerebrospinal fluid that protects your spinal cord and brain. At the time of this writing, reports are circulating about a professional boxer who died of a cerebral hemorrhage following a fight. It has been speculated that this may have been the result of crash dieting prior to weighing in. This could have contributed to severe dehydration, thus leaving the brain more vulnerable. It is also not the first correlation in the boxing world between dehydration and death due to cerebral hemorrhage.

Let this be a warning to all of you competitors considering unhealthy ways of making weight. These include saunas and steam rooms, hot showers, fluid restriction, laxatives, diuretics, and vomiting. More benign consequences may include decreased performance and heat intolerance. On the other end of the spectrum, such practices can be dangerous and perhaps fatal.

Water and Performance

Is it any wonder, then, with all the things water does for us, that a less then optimal hydration status may result in less than optimal athletic performance? Research has established this. A 2 to 4% decrease in hydration status (by body weight) can sabotage strength-training performance by 21% and aerobic performance by 48%. Dehydration can also mess with your mental sharpness. A 2% decrease in fluid status can wipe out your short-term memory and visual abilities by 20%. Not something you want to happen when someone else is trying to hit you.

Immune Function and Disease Prevention

If all of this hasn't convinced you of water's importance, consider that athletes are at increased risk for upper respiratory tract infections (URTIs), and that proper hydration status can decrease that risk. It has been shown that athletes during heavy training exhibit low levels of salivary flow and have decreased levels of antibacterial immunoglobulins in their saliva. In studies, well-hydrated athletes, and particularly those who consumed a carbohydrate beverage, had higher salivary flow and higher levels of protective immunoglobulins.

While the exact mechanism is not yet known, it appears that water plays a role in preventing more serious diseases as well. Studies have shown that low water intake may result in increased risk for colon, bladder, prostate, and kidney cancers. Researchers speculate that greater amounts of fluid accelerate the flushing away of harmful substances such as carcinogens, giving them less time in your body to do harm.

Staying Ahead of the Eight Ball

Most sedentary folks need at least 8 cups of water a day. That's just to replenish insensible water loss. "Insensible" means we don't even notice we are losing water. Water vapor is lost when we inspire air. To a certain extent, perspiration occurs without our even noticing. Water is also lost to metabolic waste products.

When we exercise, however, we sweat to keep our core temperature constant despite an increase in heat production. And we can lose a heck of a lot of water through sweat. Factors like size (surface area), sex, weather, and humidity determine the amount of water lost as sweat. Well-trained athletes may develop a more efficient cooling system and may sweat more. In humid weather, the water on your skin does not evaporate as well, so the body compensates by producing more sweat. Hot weather also adds to the burden of keeping your core temperature down. It's not surprising then, that athletes can lose up to 3 liters of water per hour! Even if the temperature is only 50°F, soccer players can lose up to 2 liters of water in 90 minutes.

You will always lose water when you exercise, and the rate at which you lose will always be greater than or equal to the rate at which you can replenish. That means you can only hope to *maintain* hydration status. If you enter a training session or event with a water deficit, you are going to be behind the eight ball no matter what you do.

One more thing about being behind the eight ball—if you fail to *fully* replenish fluids after a workout, you'll be in bad shape for the next one, and even worse shape for the one after that. That water deficit just snowballs and further compromises your performance.

The Thirst Mechanism: A Faulty Gauge

Athletes often fail to drink enough fluids simply because they simply don't feel thirsty. The problem is that the thirst mechanism only kicks in once you're already depleted by 1.5 to 2 liters. It's triggered by changes in sodium and chloride concentrations, but by the time these changes are detected, it's already too late. The trick is to drink fluids so that you won't feel thirsty in the first place.

Signs of Dehydration

Beyond thirst, how do you know when you're really dehydrated? Below is a list of common symptoms.

• Dark-colored urine	• Cough
• Cramps	• Dizziness
• Nausea and vomiting	• Gastrointestinal distress
• Loss of appetite	• Cessation of sweat
• Chills	• Painful urination
• Fatigue	• Unsteady gait
• Headache	• Increased pulse rate
• Dry mouth	• Delirium

What to Drink

Unless you're exercising for more than an hour to 90 minutes, water is your best bet. If you are exercising for over an hour, then for reasons stated in the carbohydrate section of this book, you will want to consume a carbohydrate sports beverage like Gatorade. This should be a 4–8% (approximately between 9.5 g to 19 g carbohydrate per 8 oz water) carbohydrate solution. Higher concentrations may actually delay the time it takes for both the fluids and carb to empty out of your stomach and get to the parts of your body that need them. If you need to replace a lot of fluid, then you may also want to dilute the sports beverage so as not to consume more carb or calories than you need.

To determine the concentration of the solution, use the following formula:

(# grams carbohydrate per 8 oz serving ÷ 240) x 100 = concentration of solution

As we already mentioned, fructose has been shown to cause gastrointestinal distress when used as a carbohydrate supplement during exercise. It is therefore advisable to use fruit juice as a fluid replacement *after* exercise and not during.

Fluid Guidelines

Recommendations for fluid intake are as follows.

Table 12. ACSM Guidelines for Fluid Intake

Prior to Exercise	Drink 2 cups 2 hours before.
	Drink 1 to 2 cups 15 minutes just before exercise.
During Exercise	Drink a minimum of 1 to 2 cups every 15 minutes.
Following Exercise	Drink 3 cups per pound of body weight lost.

To determine how much to drink after exercise, weigh yourself before your workout or event. After exercise, weigh yourself again (minus any wet or damp clothing) to determine how much weight in water you've lost. For each pound of weight lost, drink 2–3 cups of water.

Eyeballing It

A more practical way to determine if your hydration status is adequate is by monitoring your urine. It should be odorless and clear or only a very faint straw color. If it is dark, has an odor, or you produce very little of it, then you need to replete your body with fluids.

Hyponatremia

For all of the concern over dehydration, the opposite problem, *overhydration*, is just as dangerous. Most common among endurance athletes—marathoners and triathletes especially—hyponatremia is defined as an abnormally low plasma sodium concentration of less than 135 millimoles per liter. Endurance athletes are not the only ones at risk for hyponatremia. Anyone taking in fluids without electrolyte replacement can overhydrate.

The fluid-electrolyte balance is crucial because if the osmotic balance across the blood-brain barrier is disrupted, water can enter the brain and cause cerebral edema and, subsequently, death. Symptoms include altered "puffiness" (edema), nausea, vomiting, headache, altered mental status, pulmonary edema, and seizures.

Hyponatremia is caused by ingestion of fluids in excess of sweat and urinary water loss. Further exacerbating the problem is the loss of sodium through sweat. We lose more sodium in sweat under extreme heat conditions and when we are less conditioned. The more acclimated and fit you are, the less sodium you will lose.

To prevent hyponatremia, you'll want to determine your sweat rate. Again, weigh yourself before and after exercise. Remember, 16 oz, or 1 pint, weighs 1 pound. So if you were to lose 3 pounds of weight after an hour of exercise, you would have lost 48 oz of fluid. While everyone loses sodium at a different rate, you'll want to replace every 8 oz of fluid with about 200 mg of sodium. This approximates sodium losses in sweat, though, again, individuals will vary. So if you replace 48 oz of fluid, you'll need to replenish your sodium as well with about 1200 mg.

You can replenish sodium levels with sports drinks, though some do not have adequate ratios of sodium to fluid, so be sure to read the label. Salt tablets are another option. You can also add salt and high sodium foods to your diet before and after lengthy training sessions and events.

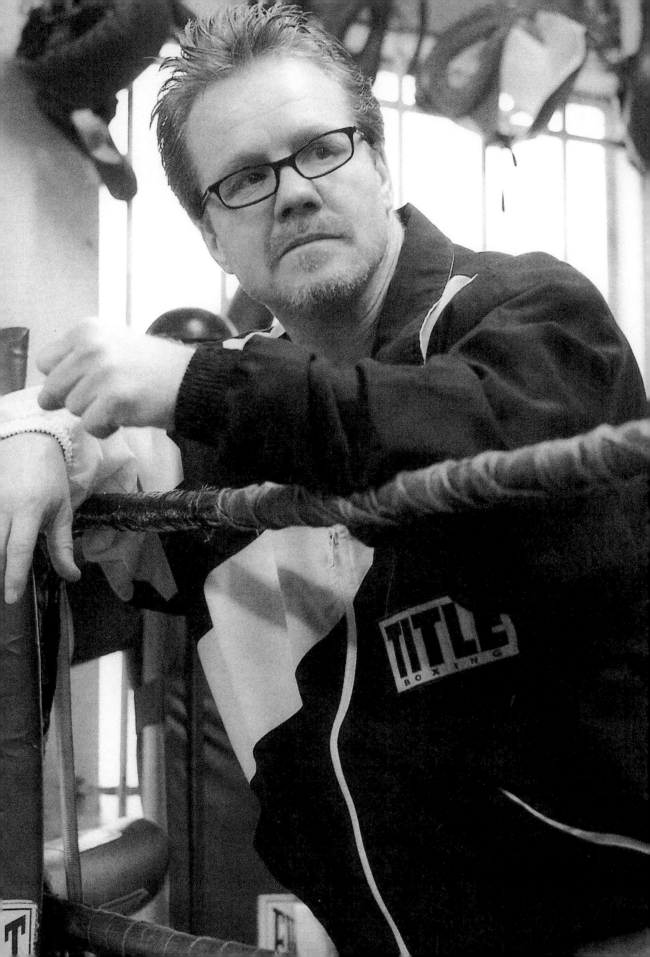

CHAPTER 17

Making Weight with Freddie Roach

Freddie Roach is one of the most respected trainers in boxing. Voted Trainer of the Year by the Boxing Writers Association of America in 2003, 2006 and 2007, he has trained the likes of Virgil Hill, James Toney, Mike Tyson, Manny Pacquiao, Oscar De La Hoya, Vladimir Klitschoko, Marlon Starling, Lucia Rijker, and Bernard Hopkins. He has already been inducted into the California Boxing Hall of Fame and the World Boxing Hall of Fame. Who better, then, to ask about the intricacies of fueling for big fights than someone who has lead his fighters to championships on the world's biggest stages?

As Freddie himself admits in this interview (conducted before I was brought on board to work with some of his fighters), boxing is still a bit in the Dark Ages when it comes to conditioning and nutrition. But as he also points out, boxing and other combat disciplines are not like other sports, and certain nutrition practices may feel uncomfortable to certain fighters when taking heavy shots to the body and head—when the intention is to knock someone unconscious. As Roach points out, there's a huge difference between the type of contact in football and fighting, and for some fighters, this adrenaline factor can make for some seemingly strange dietary practices. Here, he sheds some light on the complex intersection between modern nutritional science, our fight-or-flight reptilian brains, cultural traditions, individual superstitions, and old-school boxing practices.

Do your fighters usually come to you in good shape?
It really just depends on the individual. When Manny Pacquiao gets here from the Philippines, he gets here to start getting ready for a fight, but he's already in good shape. He's always working toward getting within striking distance. And then we have James Toney who comes in really out of shape and by fight time he gets in about halfway shape.

How well do your fighters take nutrition instruction?
Most take direction pretty well, but then you've got a veteran like James Toney who's his own man. He does what he wants. I can help guide him through things but it's ultimately his choice. Like anyone—it's ultimately their choice. The younger guys are a lot more receptive.

What are the most common adjustments you make to your fighters' diets?
I used to try to come up with the perfect formula to get a fighter ready for a world title fight. I had both Virgil Hill and Marlon Starling in the same training camp—both fighting on separate shows, though. A welterweight title fight for Marlon and a light heavyweight title fight for Virgil. I wrote down what they did everyday and the contrast was so huge, that it just didn't work. There's no actual formula for that because everyone's an individual and that's how you really have to treat them. Virgil needed to run 10 miles a day. Marlon needed to run one hour a day—not quite as fast as Virgil, though. One guy needed this. The other guy needed that. I used to keep track of that everyday for all my fighters and I stopped doing that because it really depends on the day and how they feel. You have to know when to push them and when to hold back a little bit. It's just a general feeling that I'll have. Like the workout today [with Pacquiao] is already done and gone. Now for tomorrow's workout, I already have an idea of what it may be but, again, maybe they come in tomorrow maybe they don't feel that well—it can vary. So, there's no set program. It's like day by day basically on how they feel, what they need to do, when to push them. Or maybe one day, the fight's getting close, you need to pull them back a little bit. We can't treat everybody the same because some people respond to things in different ways.

You've also talked about the mental component to training.

Yes, Virgil was such a great athlete and a great runner he used to have to run 10 miles a day. And then one day before the fight, I'd have to let him go 20. Just to get his mindset. If he didn't do that 20 that one day, he would mentally be destroyed. He just had to get that in somewhere, so somewhere along the line on a Saturday when he'd have an off day the next day, I'd have to go and let him go that 20. Marlon Starling, who I had at the same time, needed to run an hour everyday but he ran at a very slow pace. He probably got 5 to 6 miles in that hour. But he needed that longevity because of his style. He needed that long grind because he wasn't a knockout artist. Most of his fights would go the distance. He'd kind of break guys down. If he did knock them out it'd be late in the fight. They all need to work, yes, but it's give and take on how far and how much.

I was talking to Brian Villoria's dad and he said they track every calorie, every gram that he takes in. I was wondering if a lot of your fighters are like that or just some.

Some. Most, no. And one thing about the fighters making weight, they know their bodies better than anybody. From the amateurs, they know how to make weight. Obviously, I think it's much better for them to make weight earlier than the last day but for the most part, most fighters make weight the last day. That's the way it goes.

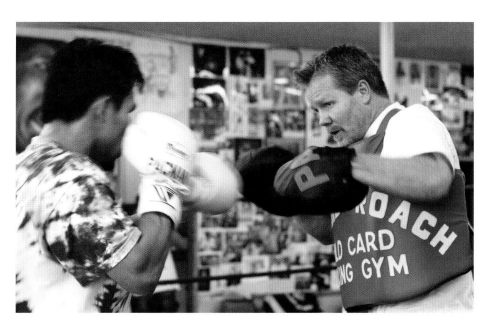

I know you've said in other interviews that you like to see your fighters make weight 3 or 4 days before, but it usually doesn't happen.
Usually doesn't happen. And you know what? It didn't even happen for me [laughs].

You've mentioned Pedialyte as a way to replenish electrolytes.
Most guys will do Pedialyte. It absorbs a little bit quicker. A lot of guys will go with Gatorade and so forth, which is not the best, because it probably has too much sugar. I think it's more mental than anything. Are they happy with it? When I used to fight, the night before a fight, I'd eat a steak. That was the thing to eat back when I fought! And I fought well. I was happy! But now it's all carbohydrates. So things have changed a little bit but for the most part boxing still isn't up to date on diet like other sports.

It's interesting, though, that you say boxing is different from other sports, so perhaps conventional sports nutrition doesn't always apply.
It is different, yes. Most strength coaches have the same idea, but it all revolves around football. For some reason, that's where they get their education because that's the biggest sport in college. But with diet, it's so different for a fighter because, again, in football, you get hit, but not like a boxer where the intention is to hit the body and head. So with my fighters, their last meal is a light meal 6 hours before the fight. It's a lot easier to rehydrate yourself nowadays because you have a 24-hour period, but when I fought, you weighed in 6 hours before a fight so we had a lot less time. And the only true way to rehydrate yourself is to get an IV, which I have done before. It's not illegal but it's just not even talked about that much, so you don't see it. But it's actually the best way to rehydrate a person. You get a nurse to stick in an IV with high glucose in it. It's a great energy boost. And I've never read anywhere that it's illegal.

Why is it that you don't hear more about IV recovery after fights?
I've used it many times. I think it's a great thing, but it's just not always available because, of course, you have to get an IV and a nurse or a doctor, you have to know somebody. My mother's a nurse, so she used to help me out. Nurses do shots way better than doctors! I think the problem is getting the IV. You've

got to know somebody in a hospital usually. Again, I don't think it's illegal and there's nothing in the IV that would test positive for an illegal drug. I've used it with James Toney. I've used it with fighters who have had trouble making weight. Just put that IV in them and they're really back to normal within a short period of time. It's the safest way to go because 90% of the stuff you take orally just comes out the other way. You're not absorbing enough of it.

For that last meal do you do any protein or is it just carbs at that point?
We've done some studies on that. We'd feed the fighter just carbs, and he'd have good explosiveness but no lasting power. And with the protein, he'd have lasting power but no explosiveness. We're pretty convinced you actually need both. So the night before a fight I like a nice fish meal for the protein and then the day of the fight you gotta go with carbohydrates, too.

And Justin Fortune didn't like to eat at all before a fight.
Justin's one of those guys. They go in the ring hungry. I had to go in with food. Because if I went in hungry, I was weak. I couldn't do it, but Justin went in hungry. And food does dull our senses a little, of course. It's like being in the service. They do all the maneuvers on an empty stomach before breakfast just because you're sharper. But the thing is, *I* couldn't do that in a fight. If you can do it, it's probably a better way to go because your senses are sharper and your reflexes are a little quicker. But with me, I'd just feel hungry and it wouldn't work.

Under normal conditions, you might pass out from low blood sugar, but I guess the adrenaline keeps you going?
Yeah, he'd be working on the meal from the night before, too. Again, every individual's different.

How much water would you take in from weigh-in until the fight?
You have a 24-hour period and they'll be sipping on it after the weigh-in and that night, and you're kind of back to normal by the next morning, or at least close. In about a 24-hour period, you're taking in 1–2 L. You'll stop about 6 hours before the fight.

Besides the steak, any other rituals?

Poached eggs and toast was my morning breakfast from when my dad was my trainer. For the most part it was the steak 6 hours before the fight. But being in the amateurs, I remember you had to weigh-in an hour before the fight. So I'd weigh in and I'd need something to eat before the fight.

I remember some fighters having soup and light stuff. I'd have a submarine sandwich. I never threw up! But I always had to have something solid in me.

Do any of your fighters have any funny rituals?

They all have little things that they do. Some things I'll notice. Some things I won't. A month before the fight, Pacquiao until the fight, nothing cold will go in his system whatsoever. He only drinks hot water, hot tea, hot milk—everything. He just has this ritual that the coldness will affect his body in a bad way.

Is that cultural?

Yes. Every fighter's superstitious because if you have a good fight, the next fight you want to do the same thing. I came in heavy one time and then I went out and lost 4 pounds to make the weight, and then I won by a third-round knockout. So the next fight I came in heavy on purpose because I thought maybe losing that 4 pounds right before the fight was good for me—and I got my ass kicked [laughs].

You didn't go back to that ritual, right?

[laughs] I didn't go back to that ritual. But my lucky shoe goes on first everyday still.

Do you recommend supplements to your clients?

Alex has the fighters on multivitamins, vitamin packets—vitamin C, stuff like that. Just to keep them healthy. Mostly it's just a high quality vitamin pack that will cover pretty much everything.

Do you mostly recommend just meat and vegetables?

Mostly. I *love* bread, so it's hard for me to stay away. But especially close to a fight, my dad made me stay away from stuff like that. I'm not used to it now because I'm not fighting anymore, but when I was fighting I would stay away from stuff like that for the most part.

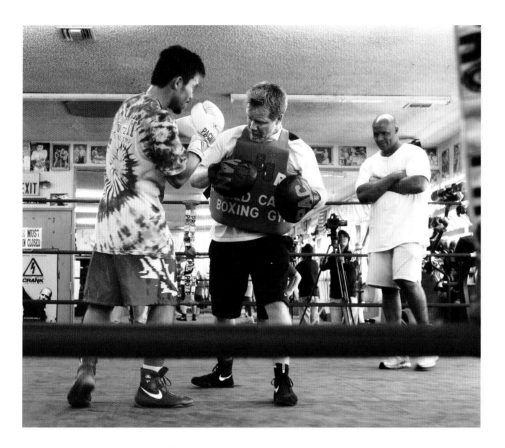

Do you include carbs earlier in the day?

Yeah, pretty much. We try not to eat any carbs after 5 pm because if you don't burn them off it just gets stored as fat. The protein will stay with you. It's better to have the carbs earlier and the protein later on. In America, we kind of eat backwards anyway. We should have the biggest meal of the day first, and our smallest last. And that's what I'm trying to do right now. Tonight I'll leave here at 8 o'clock and I'll have a salad because I'm getting too fat, so I'm just trying to be healthy.

What role do you think diet plays in your fighters' performance?

It's probably more important than a lot of people realize but, again, boxing's still not as far along as other sports. In track, they monitor their athletes a lot better than we do and boxing's still a bit in the Dark Ages. Again, if we could be around them everyday and cook for them everyday that would be the ideal situation but that's not always available. Diet is important not just for the fight, but also in getting ready for the fight—for staying healthy along the way.

CHAPTER 18

The Big Picture with Sensei Peter Freedman

Sensei Peter Freedman is the founder of Freedman's Method of Ketsugo Jujutsu. He has over 43 years of experience in the martial arts and has provided instruction in his art to law enforcement, sky marshals, the Department of Defense, the Special Forces, and the CIA. His teaching methods have saved countless lives on the streets of Boston, and the Mayor of Boston has recognized Sensei Freedman for his invaluable contributions to the community. Here, Freedman explains his no-nonsense approach to nutrition and its part in comprehensive, holistic martial arts training.[34]

I've noticed on your website you have a reading list that includes a number of nutrition books. Is this something you consider integral to the martial arts?
Most people when they teach martial arts they only teach all the techniques. They teach sparring. But if you don't have the energy if you don't eat right, if you don't have the good diet and get the proper rest, how're you supposed to focus your mind and pay attention? So I like to educate my students about the proper foods to eat, what they should be eating. And by doing this, they don't get sick and they're able to train longer and train harder. When I was going to tae kwon do school in the 1970s my instructor would *never* mention anything about nutrition. My nutrition was really bad. I was basically drinking Cokes and eating Ring Dings. Then I would go to tae kwon do school and I wasn't even drinking water! I would just drink soda. When I was thirsty I'd just

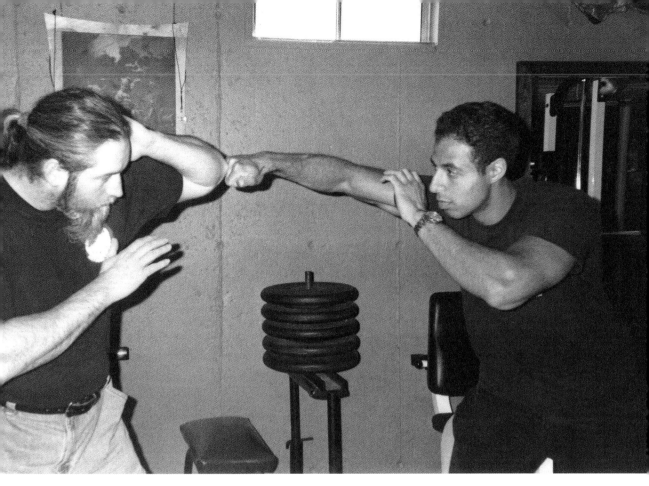

Peter Freedman training third-degree
black belt Dave Weinberg.

drink soda, which you know is worse. I would get lightheaded during training.
I'd start seeing spots before my eyes. Sometimes I'd almost faint and I didn't
know why. My teachers in martial arts never, ever stressed the importance
of nutrition. If you're eating well and you're drinking a lot of water and your
muscles are well hydrated and you work out, you heal faster, and you have
more energy. It also keeps your body fat and cholesterol down.

How do you go about educating your students on nutrition?
One of the first things I do—I do this with the kids, the teenagers, and the
adults—I teach them about water and how to constantly hydrate all day
because just through sweating and urinating and breathing, you lose a lot
of water. Water's important for keeping the skin and joints healthy and for
keeping the brain functioning properly. It helps keep the immune system up.
It helps keep down swelling in the body. Water is number one. Then, second,
I teach food, how vegetables are very important to keep bad cholesterol

down with fiber, which cleans the bile and takes the bad cholesterol out of the body. Everybody eats fiber but nobody knows why they have to. If I teach them how fiber works it's easier for people to want to eat it. Then I teach them how not to overeat carbohydrates because carbohydrates turn to body fat. I make people read books and self-educate so they retain it better. It helps them to take part in their own health.

Third, I teach sleep, which helps with digestion, and you should never eat directly before going to bed. Some people, if they're doing chi kung and meditate, they only need 5 or 6 hours of sleep because of their chi kung training. A person not meditating probably needs 7 or 8. Your body charges itself between 10 at night until 5 o'clock in the morning. And then it stops around 5:30 to 6 o'clock. And that's why all the tai chi masters get up at 5 and do all their tai chi and chi kung early in the morning. There's a magnetic pull of the planet. The other planets affect the magnetic pull. During the nighttime hours the magnetic pull of the planet is recharging the body, but your body can't accept the charge unless you're sleeping. That's why people do chi kung— to give themselves more energy so they use less of their life energy. Going to bed late and waking up late drains your chi. That's why it's good to get up early. It'll increase your health, your immune system. It'll give you more strength.

If you go to bed late, your body is under duress. By going to bed late and getting up late, your body thinks it's under stress and you start storing fat. That's from the caveman days.

It's not just nutrition; that's why I say sleep is important. Water, nutrition, and sleep. Most bad backs and lower back pain come from lack of water. As soon as you wake up, you should force yourself to drink two glasses of water. And then continue sipping water throughout the day. You're breathing deep all night, so you're losing water. If you're dehydrated, it ruins your joints and if you start hitting stuff, you're going to have problems. Plus if you're working out and sweating, you should be putting water back in your body. So that's why I teach water first, nutrition second, and sleep third. If you're getting plenty of water, and you're eating 5 to 6 times a day and it's good food, you will be able to sleep soundly. But if you're not drinking water and your food isn't right, you're going to have disturbed sleep.

I think every martial artist should know about nutrition because without nutrition your martial art isn't going to go far.

Do you have specific ratios you recommend?

I don't give my students a general nutrition plan because everyone's got to find their own. Some people may need more carb, less protein. Some people may need more protein, less carbs, and more fat. Everybody's combination is different.

There's a book on your reading list about healing teas. Can you elaborate?

When I used to study Kung Fu back in the 1970s I went to 2 or 3 schools at the same time and at one of the schools, my sifu had three types of healing teas. I think one was called shiu wu chi. It builds up the blood. When you're pounding your hands and whacking your arms, kicking the bag, you're building bruises on the inside. And they have an ointment, a tonic that goes on the outside of the body called dit dao jao. This would keep the bruising down and keep the bones healthy by keeping the blood down. And then when you would drink the shiu wu chi that would make the blood stronger and prevent you from bruising on the inside.

The other two teas, I don't know—I think the first tea was jasmine. One of them was to build up chi in the body and it would actually make you healthier. He had it shipped in from China in the 70s. The chi would help the body heal for the next training session. When I was going there I had a lot of energy. It was amazing. I saw a student there who came in with a cast on his arm with a compound break. That's when the bone comes through the skin. He had to go and have his arm reset and stitched up and sifu cut the cast off. I couldn't believe it; the kid was freaked out. *I* was freaked out. And he put medicine where the stitches were and within a day or two it was completely healed, and he could pull the stitches out. Then he put another medicine on his arm that made the bones heal for one and a half weeks. And within the second week, the guy was whacking his arms against the post. Now you know if you break your arm, it's four to six weeks. And this guy was whacking his arms and lifting weights with his arms in two weeks.

When you trained with this sifu he taught you all about the herbs, about the teas, how to make your own medicine. We all had to sit down and write notes. He would teach us the history of the art. But back then I was more interested in fighting, because I was getting into fights every single day on the streets. I was in knife fights, stick fights, gang fights. I had people shooting at me. I had people hunting me. I had to look over my shoulder all the time. I wanted to learn how to fight, fight, fight. That's all I cared about, because I needed it.

So I didn't stick with him long enough. I was a fool. Because he was only charging 15 dollars a month, 3 days a week. These guys could actually snap wood off a 2-by-4. He had special herbs that you would put on your skin; the average person with a strong grip would rip their skin off but not these guys. He also had herbs to make the tendons and ligaments stronger. I tried to go back and train with him, but he had moved away.

You don't really hear about these things in modern dojos. Do you think these traditions are gradually being lost?

I think a lot of those traditions are already lost. There are keepers of the knowledge like that but like with my art of jujutsu, I had to go outside of jujutsu and do research and study with other people and other arts to learn their concepts and principles, to put back in my jujutsu what has been missing. I'm going to be doing that for the rest of my life.

You used to be a power lifter, right?

People always say you should never lift weights when you're doing martial arts. But I believe some people need to lift weights. They're too weak, too skinny. It depends on the individual. I was a power lifter. My nutrition changed, because the guy who taught me power lifting did 3 or 4 tours in Korea, did a couple of tours in Vietnam. This guy was no joke. He was also a respiratory therapist. He knew everything about the anatomy and nutrition—he was a walking encyclopedia. He said, "Pete, if you're a power lifter, you've got to eat the right foods." I didn't know that. So he started teaching me about nutrition. I started reading every single book I could get my hands on.

Do you eat organic?

My friend Chick Weatherbee is a naturopath, and he'll tell me to cut out all processed foods. And the only foods you can eat have to be organic. He'll say if you have a choice of eating a carrot that's not organic or not eating the carrot at all, don't eat the carrot at all. Because carrots are roots. The carrots absorb the chemicals in the ground. The problem is organic food is so damn expensive. I think that's a trick to keep everybody sick. The drug companies run the government. They run the FDA. If people get healthy, then the drug companies won't make any money. There are a lot of doctors who prescribe to their patients drugs they would never take themselves.

Do you take any supplements?
I stopped completely because a lot of them trigger my asthma. I think I'm allergic to the bonding agents and some of the fillers. A lot of people don't know about the fillers—people are allergic to those fillers, and that's why I've got asthma. I found that I'm better off just juicing vegetables.

Everyone should get a juicer. Don't buy pre-made juices. You've got to make your own. Pre-made juices are dead food. You want to eat live food. You get carrots, you get celery, you get beets. Those juice books have recipes for every illness, and they work! You've got to stick with them and stop eating the junk. A lot of people can't afford to stop eating the junk because if you stop eating the junk, you get sick. Your body will have withdrawal. You've got to slowly come off the junk food. It's like a drug.

Now they do have good quality vitamins out there, but you've got to do your research and find out what the binding agents are that are holding the vitamins together. You may be allergic to them and they'll trigger an allergic reaction. Some of these companies' vitamins have molds from the nuts in them. There's a really popular brand that I read the label for one time, and they had an allowance for rat droppings and they also put in shellac. I think they were also putting in sawdust. Just as fillers so they could make it and get it out there in large quantities. And everybody's buying [this brand].

Some people do need vitamins if you're not getting it in your food. But if you have a choice between a pill and juicing, I would say juice, because you don't get the fillers and bonding agents. Carrots and celery are really good. That's what my teacher always drank. You've got to be careful about beets. They're really good for you, because they're alkaline in your body. But when you go to the bathroom, you'll think you're dying! The first time my teacher told me to do beets, I called him up and thought that I was dying…I put my things in order and thought that I was really dying [laughs]. But that's just the beet juice. If you get a juicer, get a good juicer, not a cheap one. I have one from Italy. It's $350, all stainless steel. My other juicers would actually walk right off the table. The Juiceman book is good.

Morihei Ueshiba once said, "Food is the a gift from the universe. No, in a sense food is the universe." Care to elaborate?

He's right on the money. If you think about it all your vegetables are from the sun. The sun is part of the universe. Plus there's energy in food. Food vibrates. Your body vibrates. The planet vibrates. The chair you sit in. The couch you lie on. Everything vibrates. When he says that food is the universe, the food you're eating is actually part of you. If you're eating any kind of vegetables or fruit you're eating the sun. If you're eating any kind of meat, you're eating the sun unless you're eating some kind of meat that was raised indoors under fluorescent lights. Even junk food is universal because it vibrates. It's just that you want to eat the good vibrational foods. That's not processed foods. Because anything that man touches is no good. Go out into the woods where it's really quiet and watch what the animals eat. If you copy what the animals eat, most of the time, you can eat that. The animals know what's good and what isn't good. Of course, some animals can eat a different kind of roughage because we don't have the appendix thing going anymore and they have shorter intestines. But everything is universal.

As some of the fighting arts have been modified to become sports, it seems there is less longevity and more injury. The traditional elderly martial arts master is becoming even more of a rarity and more so here than in other countries.

A martial artist should be a trained warrior. He should go beyond the athlete. An athlete trains for competition. A martial artist trains for life. An athlete's training for his career. A martial artist trains for the rest of his life.

Professional athletes are training more. All their joints are messed up. They age faster. They're agitated. They're angry, depressed. But a martial artist, as they get older, they're like a fine wine. They become better. Bruce Lee was getting better as he was getting older. Look at O Sensei, Ueshiba, he could just toss people around in his old age. On his deathbed he threw two of his students across the room! He tried to get up and they went to help him and he threw them across the room. Now let's get an athlete who's 60 years old and see if the athlete can keep up with the young people. He can't. But a martial artist can.

Over here it's fast everything. Everybody wants a black belt in one month. Everybody wants all the techniques. What's happening is martial arts have become a business. A lot of people are afraid of getting sued and they don't have the same knowledge they had then for dealing with safety and health issues.

In other martial arts schools here, nobody's doing that—nobody's educating students about anatomy or nutrition. How can you do martial arts without nutrition? In other countries they educate. Why not in this country? I just don't understand why it's not being done here. I have some people who are sick and come to me for Reiki, and I tell them if they change their diet, they won't be sick. And they say, "No, no, no—I'll just take a pill." So they take medication but they could get off the medication if they start eating right. But they'd rather *not* eat right and take the pill. That's the mentality of most of the country. That's why this country is in trouble right now. I don't know what's going to happen, but people need to wake up. You've got to take responsibility for your own body. If you want to be a good fighter it all starts with drinking water, eating right, and sleep. And *then* training.

Freedman training third-degree black belt Dave Weinberg.

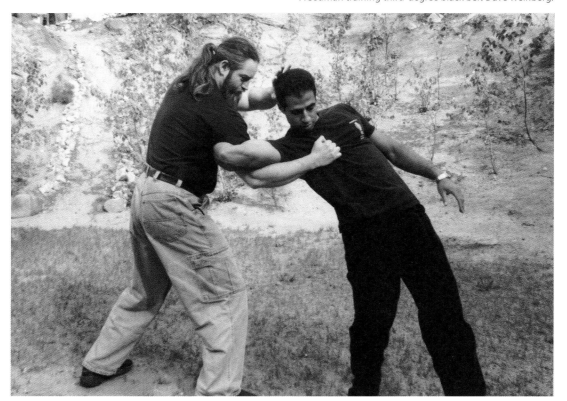

CHAPTER 19

Real-World Progress: Case Files

As we said at the beginning of this book, all the information and strategies in the world aren't going to get you results. You must *execute*. Zen *is* experience, not some philosophy that exists in a test tube. I can't give you that actual experience in a book, but I can do the next best thing—give you a few stories and examples of those who have followed the strategies explained here and have experienced amazing results.

These client success stories range from the more down-to-earth examples—a police detective whose life depends on his fitness, and a competitive athlete whose triathlon performance reflects her nutrition/training balance—to the approaches used by champion-level martial artists Khan, Pacquiao, and Arlovski. In each case, you'll see some of the potential obstacles you yourself may face and how we dealt with them. You'll see everything we've discussed so far put into practice. This will give you an idea of how to navigate through the program yourself and what to expect.

To record client progress, I use What Works Nutrition Software® which is the best software of its kind. At the bottom half of each chart, you'll see four graphs. From the top left graph moving clockwise, these graphs represent body fat percentage, weight, muscle loss/gain, and fat loss/gain. You can find out more about this software at www.WhatWorksNutritionSoftware.com.

Street-Smart Eating

"As a detective in South East LA, I work long unusual hours. Eating was usually on the fly and sporadic at best. My job requires me to deal with people—mostly LA gangsters—on the streets. I'm in vehicle pursuits, foot chases and physical altercations daily, so fitness and nutrition are very important to me.

"Anyone who weight trains regularly knows how hard it is to increase muscle mass. When I started with Teri, I was 5'8", 143.5 pounds, and 6.14% body fat. Not bad, but I felt it could be better. As of my last session, I am 150 pounds and 4.46% body fat. Don't let Teri's mild mannered demeanor fool you. She plays no games and pulls no punches. She will tell it to you like it is, but is very positive and knowledgeable about what she does. My gains would have been impossible without her. She guided me step by step and it paid off. As long as you have the dedication to do what she says, you will absolutely, positively meet your physical goals."

—Brett Benson, SIU Detective, Gang Investigations

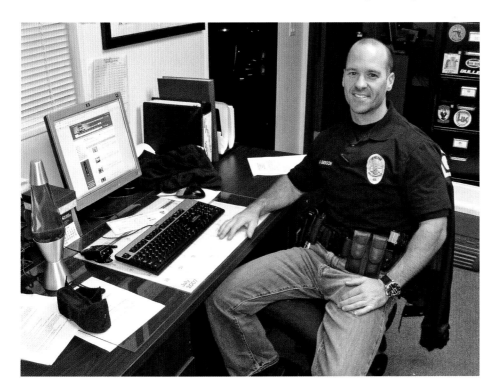

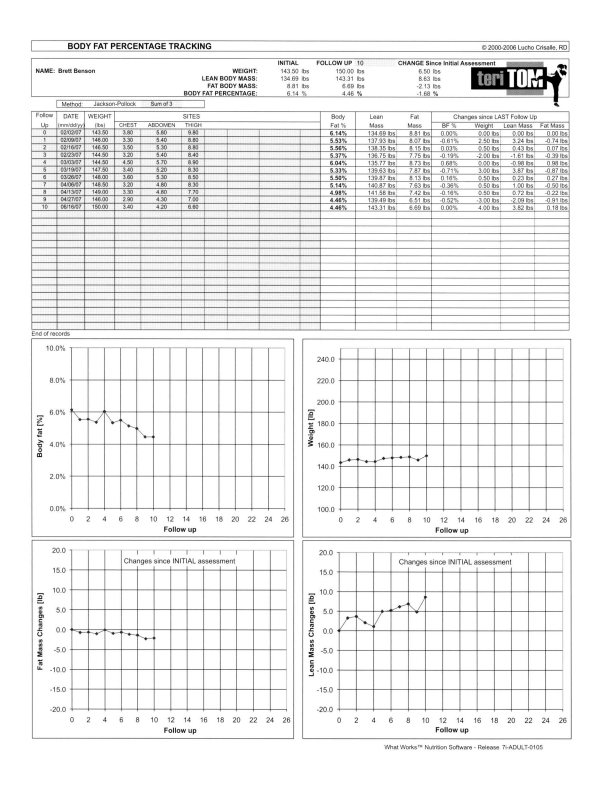

BODY FAT PERCENTAGE TRACKING

© 2000-2006 Lucho Crisalle, RD

NAME: Brett Benson

	INITIAL	FOLLOW UP 10	CHANGE Since Initial Assessment
WEIGHT:	143.50 lbs	150.00 lbs	6.50 lbs
LEAN BODY MASS:	134.69 lbs	143.31 lbs	8.63 lbs
FAT BODY MASS:	8.81 lbs	6.69 lbs	-2.13 lbs
BODY FAT PERCENTAGE:	6.14 %	4.46 %	-1.68 %

Method: Jackson-Pollock   Sum of 3

Follow Up	DATE (mm/dd/yy)	WEIGHT (lbs)	SITES CHEST	ABDOMEN	THIGH	Body Fat %	Lean Mass	Fat Mass	Changes since LAST Follow Up BF %	Weight	Lean Mass	Fat Mass
0	02/02/07	143.50	3.80	5.80	9.80	**6.14%**	134.69 lbs	8.81 lbs	0.00%	0.00 lbs	0.00 lbs	0.00 lbs
1	02/09/07	146.00	3.30	5.40	8.80	**5.53%**	137.93 lbs	8.07 lbs	-0.61%	2.50 lbs	3.24 lbs	-0.74 lbs
2	02/16/07	146.50	3.50	5.30	8.80	**5.56%**	138.35 lbs	8.15 lbs	0.03%	0.50 lbs	0.43 lbs	0.07 lbs
3	02/23/07	144.50	3.20	5.40	8.40	**5.37%**	136.75 lbs	7.75 lbs	-0.19%	-2.00 lbs	-1.61 lbs	-0.39 lbs
4	03/03/07	144.50	4.50	5.70	8.90	**6.04%**	135.77 lbs	8.73 lbs	0.68%	0.00 lbs	-0.98 lbs	0.98 lbs
5	03/19/07	147.50	3.40	5.20	8.30	**5.33%**	139.63 lbs	7.87 lbs	-0.71%	3.00 lbs	3.87 lbs	-0.87 lbs
6	03/26/07	148.00	3.60	5.30	8.50	**5.50%**	139.87 lbs	8.13 lbs	0.16%	0.50 lbs	0.23 lbs	0.27 lbs
7	04/06/07	148.50	3.20	4.80	8.30	**5.14%**	140.87 lbs	7.63 lbs	-0.36%	0.50 lbs	1.00 lbs	-0.50 lbs
8	04/13/07	149.00	3.30	4.80	7.70	**4.98%**	141.58 lbs	7.42 lbs	-0.16%	0.50 lbs	0.72 lbs	-0.22 lbs
9	04/27/07	146.00	2.90	4.30	7.00	**4.46%**	139.49 lbs	6.51 lbs	-0.52%	-3.00 lbs	-2.09 lbs	-0.91 lbs
10	06/16/07	150.00	3.40	4.20	6.60	**4.46%**	143.31 lbs	6.69 lbs	0.00%	4.00 lbs	3.82 lbs	0.18 lbs

End of records

What Works™ Nutrition Software - Release 7i-ADULT-0105

Brett's story is probably closest to the spirit of this book. While I do believe food should be enjoyed, eating is also for survival so that our bodies are functioning optimally. This is obvious if you are an athlete training for performance, but it's even more crucial when your life depends on it on the streets.

When Brett showed up at my office, he was already in excellent condition. He was looking to put on a little more muscle so that he would be strong for his new gig in the Special Investigations Unit. Upon looking at his intake, I made two major changes. First, he needed to eat on a regular schedule. Because of his irregular schedule, he was going a lot longer than 4 hours between meals—sometimes, 6, 7, or 8 hours. In order for him to put on any more muscle, we had to make sure his body wasn't cannibalizing his own lean tissue. The second change was in giving him much more protein than he had been taking in. Not only was his own body eating away at his muscle, he didn't have enough of the raw material to build new muscle. We more than doubled his intake of high quality protein which included lean turkey, fish, chicken, steak, and egg whites. To make things easy for those times when his schedule would become erratic, we included protein supplements that he could conveniently drink if there was no time for real food. We fiddled a little with the protein numbers and settled at about 3,000 calories for his daily energy intake.

You'll see in weeks 3 and 4 he lost a little muscle as he was adjusting to his new job and schedule. He skipped a few meals and lost about 2 pounds of muscle in those weeks. It was smooth sailing until week 9 when he ran a race in Vegas. In the heat of competition (and the desert air), he was operating mostly in anaerobic mode and, as we expected, he dropped 2 pounds of muscle there.

In the next month, though, he put that weight back on by going back to the eating plan and his regular lifting and cardio programs. At 5'8", he now weighs 150 pounds, his highest weight ever, and 4.46% body fat. Since we started this plan, he is up 8.63 pounds in muscle and down 1.68% body fat.

At this point, it's important to note that Brett's decided to maintain at 150. To gain any more weight, even though it would be muscle and he might be stronger, would slow him down. Always know what you want to accomplish with any nutrition or exercise plan. In this case, Brett knew he wanted to be stronger without sacrificing speed. More of anything—be it muscle, weight loss, cardio—is not always necessarily better. Be sure to consider all the other variables and how to best balance them.

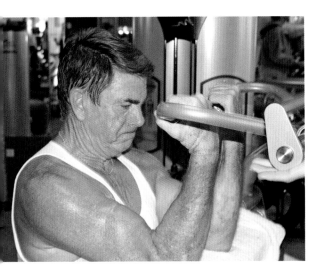

The 4000-kCal "Diet": You Are the Creator of Your Metabolism

"Since I started this project, I am down 40 pounds, my pants are down from 40 to 32" waist, and my shirt size is down from large to medium (down from 16/34-35 to 15 ½ /32-33). My body fat is down from 32.08% to 9.94%. That's progress, and a bit expensive (new clothes)! Thank you, Teri."

—Jim McCashin

Jim's chart is one of my favorites to show new clients because it gives them a very good idea of how their plans may have to change over time and why weekly monitoring is so important. Jim first weighed in at 216 and 32.08% body fat. The second follow-up, we measured him at 21.59% body fat and 217 pounds. I tell my clients that usually, the first week we are looking at some water loss that comes with a change in macronutrient ratios—often caused by a dramatic decrease in carbs. You won't, for example, lose 23 pounds of fat or gain 23 pounds of muscle in a week. The water loss that first week affects the caliper numbers and, therefore, throws off all the other numbers.

I tell clients to look at the second follow-up as our new baseline. Also notice that Jim went up a half pound the first week as well. This is not uncommon. Often, clients who have been used to eating sporadically may put on a little muscle the first week because for the first time, they are eating in a way (sufficient protein and at 3–4 hour intervals) that supports muscle building. In this case, though, it was probably because Jim had come in with no food in him for the first follow up. Remember a measly pint weighs a pound, so your weight can fluctuate wildly throughout the day just based on the amount of food and fluids you have in you. You can see why weight isn't such a great number for assessing progress.

From week two, it was smooth sailing until week five, when Jim lost both fat and muscle. Remember from our four scenarios, that if this is the case, we increase protein. So we did. It happened again the next four weeks and in week 11 as well. We gradually increased the protein each time.

BODY FAT PERCENTAGE TRACKING

© 2000-2005 Lucho Crisalle, RD

NAME: Jim McCashin

	INITIAL	FOLLOW UP 26	CHANGE Since Initial Assessment
WEIGHT:	216.50 lbs	193.00 lbs	-23.50 lbs
LEAN BODY MASS:	147.05 lbs	173.07 lbs	26.03 lbs
FAT BODY MASS:	69.45 lbs	19.93 lbs	-49.53 lbs
BODY FAT PERCENTAGE:	32.08 %	10.32 %	-21.76 %

EXERCISE & NUTRITION

Method: Jackson-Pollock Sum of 3

Follow Up	DATE (mm/dd/yy)	WEIGHT (lbs)	SITES CHEST	ABDOMEN	THIGH	Body Fat %	Lean Mass	Fat Mass	Changes since LAST Follow Up BF %	Weight	Lean Mass	Fat Mass
0	07/11/05	216.50	27.20	35.60	37.10	32.08%	147.05 lbs	69.45 lbs	0.00%	0.00 lbs	0.00 lbs	0.00 lbs
1	07/18/05	217.00	16.20	28.20	15.50	21.59%	170.15 lbs	46.85 lbs	-10.49%	0.50 lbs	23.10 lbs	-22.60 lbs
2	07/25/05	212.50	13.90	25.90	12.80	19.48%	171.11 lbs	41.39 lbs	-2.11%	-4.50 lbs	0.96 lbs	-5.46 lbs
3	08/01/05	212.00	10.90	23.80	11.70	17.64%	174.60 lbs	37.40 lbs	-1.84%	-0.50 lbs	3.49 lbs	-3.99 lbs
4	08/10/05	210.00	8.20	21.10	11.50	15.95%	176.51 lbs	33.49 lbs	-1.69%	-2.00 lbs	1.91 lbs	-3.91 lbs
5	08/15/05	206.50	7.20	20.30	10.90	15.21%	175.09 lbs	31.41 lbs	-0.74%	-3.50 lbs	-1.42 lbs	-2.08 lbs
6	08/22/05	204.50	7.60	18.30	10.40	14.56%	174.72 lbs	29.78 lbs	-0.65%	-2.00 lbs	-0.37 lbs	-1.63 lbs
7	08/29/05	204.00	7.40	18.30	10.70	14.59%	174.23 lbs	29.77 lbs	0.03%	-0.50 lbs	-0.49 lbs	-0.01 lbs
8	09/07/05	199.50	7.00	17.20	9.90	13.88%	171.81 lbs	27.69 lbs	-0.71%	-4.50 lbs	-2.42 lbs	-2.08 lbs
9	09/15/05	199.50	6.20	16.60	9.90	13.44%	172.69 lbs	26.81 lbs	-0.44%	0.00 lbs	0.87 lbs	-0.87 lbs
10	09/21/05	199.50	6.30	16.20	10.10	13.41%	172.75 lbs	26.75 lbs	-0.03%	0.00 lbs	0.06 lbs	-0.06 lbs
11	09/26/05	194.00	6.20	15.10	9.10	12.72%	169.33 lbs	24.67 lbs	-0.69%	-5.50 lbs	-3.42 lbs	-2.08 lbs
12	10/03/05	194.50	6.20	15.90	9.70	13.16%	168.91 lbs	25.59 lbs	0.44%	0.50 lbs	-0.42 lbs	0.92 lbs
13	10/12/05	196.00	5.60	15.00	9.50	12.62%	171.26 lbs	24.74 lbs	-0.54%	1.50 lbs	2.35 lbs	-0.85 lbs
14	10/17/05	192.00	5.10	14.10	9.20	12.08%	168.80 lbs	23.20 lbs	-0.54%	-4.00 lbs	-2.46 lbs	-1.54 lbs
15	10/24/05	194.00	5.50	13.20	9.60	12.05%	170.62 lbs	23.38 lbs	-0.03%	2.00 lbs	1.82 lbs	0.18 lbs
16	11/01/05	193.50	5.50	12.10	9.10	11.54%	171.16 lbs	22.34 lbs	-0.51%	-0.50 lbs	0.55 lbs	-1.05 lbs
17	11/07/05	193.00	5.70	12.90	9.40	11.96%	169.92 lbs	23.08 lbs	0.41%	-0.50 lbs	-1.24 lbs	0.74 lbs
18	11/17/05	193.00	5.40	12.70	8.30	11.45%	170.91 lbs	22.09 lbs	-0.51%	0.00 lbs	0.98 lbs	-0.98 lbs
19	11/23/05	194.00	5.40	11.40	8.60	11.13%	172.41 lbs	21.59 lbs	-0.32%	1.00 lbs	1.51 lbs	-0.51 lbs
20	11/30/05	195.50	5.50	11.90	9.20	11.51%	173.00 lbs	22.50 lbs	0.38%	1.50 lbs	0.58 lbs	0.92 lbs
21	12/08/05	192.50	5.00	10.60	8.80	10.81%	171.70 lbs	20.80 lbs	-0.70%	-3.00 lbs	-1.30 lbs	-1.70 lbs
22	12/15/05	193.00	5.30	10.20	8.30	10.61%	172.51 lbs	20.49 lbs	-0.19%	0.50 lbs	0.82 lbs	-0.32 lbs
23	12/22/05	193.50	4.80	10.30	8.50	10.55%	173.09 lbs	20.41 lbs	-0.06%	0.50 lbs	0.57 lbs	-0.07 lbs
24	01/05/06	192.50	4.30	10.40	8.10	10.29%	172.69 lbs	19.81 lbs	-0.26%	-1.00 lbs	-0.40 lbs	-0.60 lbs
25	01/12/06	191.00	4.70	10.10	7.90	10.26%	171.40 lbs	19.60 lbs	-0.03%	-1.50 lbs	-1.28 lbs	-0.22 lbs
26	01/19/06	193.00	4.80	10.70	7.40	10.32%	173.07 lbs	19.93 lbs	0.06%	2.00 lbs	1.67 lbs	0.33 lbs

End of records

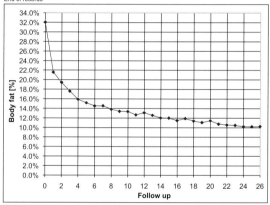

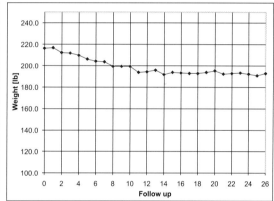

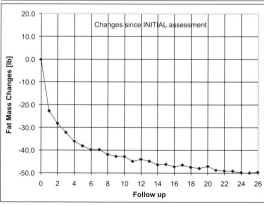

Changes since INITIAL assessment

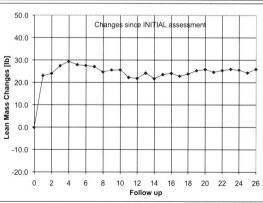

Changes since INITIAL assessment

Personal Trainer - Release 7i-ADULT-0105

Then in week 12, Jim actually lost muscle and gained fat. Remember that in this scenario, we increase calories overall, which we did by about 300 calories. Things went well until week 17 when we had to increase calories by another 300. Also notice that in week 20, both fat and muscle went *up*. This is indicative of too many calories, so we scaled back. And then the next week, Jim lost both muscle and fat, so we had to increase protein. We also did this in weeks 24 and 25.

I love to show Jim's chart to new clients because it provides excellent examples of how we constantly need to adjust your plan as your body composition changes. As Jim became leaner, he needed more and more calories. If he had, for example, not come in for a body composition assessment in week 17, we wouldn't have known what was happening. He would have continued losing muscle and gaining fat. If he'd skipped four weeks in a row, he may have spent four weeks going in the wrong direction! By monitoring body composition changes weekly, you can catch bumps in the road early and correct them. This will get you to your goals in the most efficient way possible.

The irony of Jim's chart is that he started at 32% body fat and 2100 calories. By the end of the chart, he's now 10% body fat on 4000 calories! And the best part of this story is that he was 63 years old when he did this. Who says we aren't the creators of our metabolism?

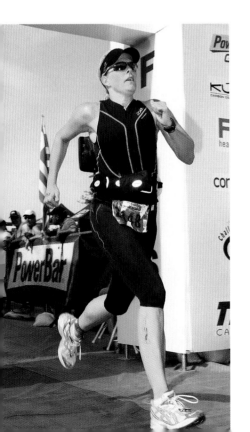

Ironwoman

"From the minute I met Teri, I knew I was in good hands. Teri has been an incredible resource for me in understanding the specific needs of my body at different activity levels. I have changed my body composition from 25% to 16% body fat and gained 10 pounds of lean muscle. Thanks to Teri's expertise and commitment, I am on my way to completing my first Ironman!"

—Kim Katz

When Kim's trainer first brought her by my office, they were stumped. She had been working out *hard*—at least two hours a

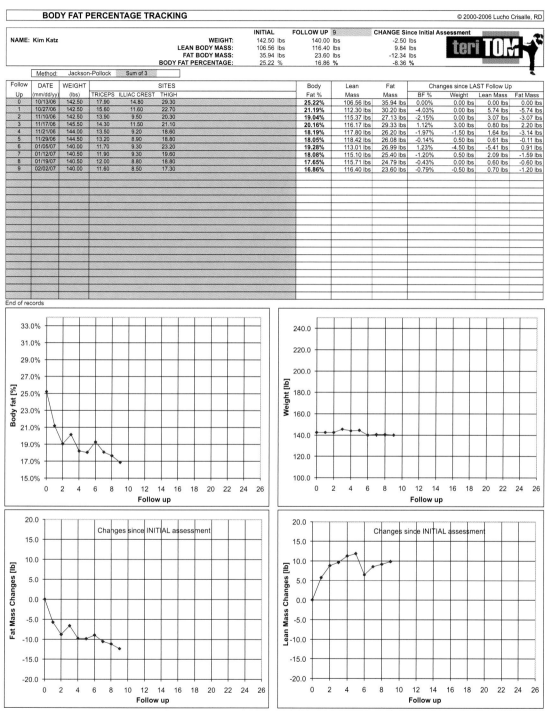

BODY FAT PERCENTAGE TRACKING

NAME: Kim Katz

	INITIAL	FOLLOW UP 9	CHANGE Since Initial Assessment
WEIGHT:	142.50 lbs	140.00 lbs	-2.50 lbs
LEAN BODY MASS:	106.56 lbs	116.40 lbs	9.84 lbs
FAT BODY MASS:	35.94 lbs	23.60 lbs	-12.34 lbs
BODY FAT PERCENTAGE:	25.22 %	16.86 %	-8.36 %

Method: Jackson-Pollock   Sum of 3

Follow Up	DATE (mm/dd/yy)	WEIGHT (lbs)	SITES TRICEPS	SITES ILLIAC CREST	SITES THIGH	Body Fat %	Lean Mass	Fat Mass	Changes since LAST Follow Up BF %	Weight	Lean Mass	Fat Mass
0	10/13/06	142.50	17.90	14.80	29.30	25.22%	106.56 lbs	35.94 lbs	0.00%	0.00 lbs	0.00 lbs	0.00 lbs
1	10/27/06	142.50	15.60	11.60	22.70	21.19%	112.30 lbs	30.20 lbs	-4.03%	0.00 lbs	5.74 lbs	-5.74 lbs
2	11/10/06	142.50	13.90	9.50	20.30	19.04%	115.37 lbs	27.13 lbs	-2.15%	0.00 lbs	3.07 lbs	-3.07 lbs
3	11/17/06	145.50	14.30	11.50	21.10	20.16%	116.17 lbs	29.33 lbs	1.12%	3.00 lbs	0.80 lbs	2.20 lbs
4	11/21/06	144.00	13.50	9.20	18.60	18.19%	117.80 lbs	26.20 lbs	-1.97%	-1.50 lbs	1.64 lbs	-3.14 lbs
5	11/29/06	144.50	13.20	8.90	18.80	18.05%	118.42 lbs	26.08 lbs	-0.14%	0.50 lbs	0.61 lbs	-0.11 lbs
6	01/05/07	140.00	11.70	9.30	23.20	19.28%	113.01 lbs	26.99 lbs	1.23%	-4.50 lbs	-5.41 lbs	0.91 lbs
7	01/12/07	140.50	11.90	9.30	19.60	18.08%	115.10 lbs	25.40 lbs	-1.20%	0.50 lbs	2.09 lbs	-1.59 lbs
8	01/19/07	140.50	12.00	8.80	18.80	17.65%	115.71 lbs	24.79 lbs	-0.43%	0.00 lbs	0.60 lbs	-0.60 lbs
9	02/02/07	140.00	11.60	8.50	17.30	16.86%	116.40 lbs	23.60 lbs	-0.79%	-0.50 lbs	0.70 lbs	-1.20 lbs

End of records

day—with her heart rate well above the 170's. "I'm working out so much," she said, "I can't understand why I'm getting fatter!" At the time, she was only doing about 1400 calories a day. We used the BodyGem™, a resting metabolic test, and found that her resting metabolic rate was actually very high—1760 calories a day.

Clearly, she wasn't getting enough food. So the first thing we did was bump her calories up to 2300. Next, she took her cardio sessions down in intensity and spent more of her time in the 140–150 BPM range with some intervals thrown in. Kim's case is one of the most common I see in my practice. She was doing what everyone intuitively thinks is right—she ate less and exercised harder. This might work for a short time, but the reason why so many people fail with their fitness plans is that they don't know how to adjust properly when they hit a plateau. Once you've been exercising for a while and have built some muscle, you need to feed that muscle. Your caloric intake actually needs to increase before your body is willing to give up any more fat. Kim was essentially in starvation mode. Her body was chomping on her lean muscle because, one, she wasn't getting enough calories, and, two, she was exercising too intensely—a real double whammy.

As you'll see from her chart, we actually had to increase her calories one more time, before she hit 16% body fat. In the sixth follow-up, notice she had put on 1 pound of fat and lost 5 pounds in muscle, so we bumped calories up another 300, which put her at a total of 2600 calories.

After coming down to 16% body fat, Kim just finished her first Ironman triathlon. We watched her composition weekly, which helped us determine her over 3,000 calorie intake. About six weeks before her event she started to feel the onset of a respiratory infection. We switched up her multivitamin to a high–quality pharmaceutical-grade brand. She went into her event without a sniffle and with her best training times.

 Throughout the entire process—either during increased training loads, tapering, competition, or during recovery—we are constantly fiddling with Kim's plan. Calories, supplements, and ratios must all be adjusted accordingly to balance both her competition and composition goals. Now that her event is over, Kim will be going back to more anaerobic exercise, including more weightlifting and some boxing. We will once again have to change her plan. As we've said throughout this book, your body is *always* changing. Your exercise and nutrition plans have to adjust to those changes.

The Fighters

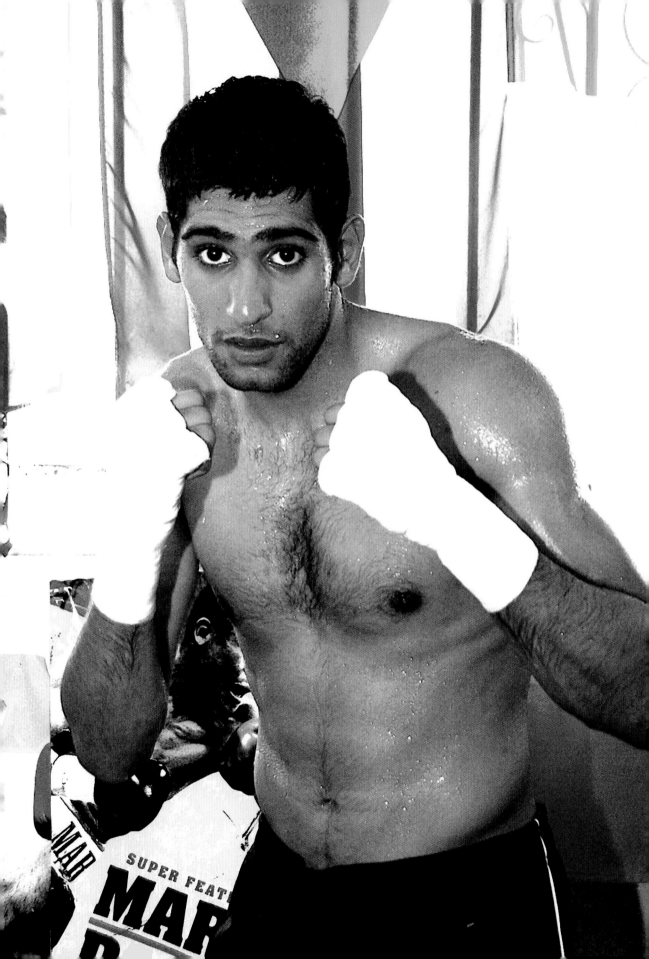

Amir Khan

Conditioning coach Alex Ariza and I started working with Amir Khan when he came to Los Angeles to work with trainer Freddie Roach. He was just coming off the only loss of his career, a devastating knockout in the first round to Brandies Prescott. In a ballsy move to turn things around, he immediately took a fight, only months afterwards. To prepare for it, he came to LA for six weeks to train with Freddie.

Obviously, he had come to Freddie for some major technical changes, but there was also a lot to do on the conditioning and body composition fronts. Amir had started out as the Olympic silver medalist in the 2004 Games. Coming out of the amateurs, he had a great jab and movement, but somewhere along the way in his pro career, he'd been given instruction to sit on his shots and move less.

To go along with this change in fighting style, he was given a workout and nutrition regimen more appropriate for bodybuilders than boxers. He was lifting very, very heavy weights. Climbing ropes with weighted vests. And like bodybuilders, he was told to do minimal cardio—only twice a week! The result of this kind of training, of course, was that he was, as they say in Britain, "massive."

When he came to Wildcard, his entire upper body, especially his back, was over-developed while his legs, were underdeveloped. Not a good combination for a boxer. Too much bulk up top limits your range of motion and reach. And worst of all, it really slows you down. Strength is different from size. In any combat sport, the muscle you put on needs to be *functional* muscle.

In designing Amir's strength program, Alex's other main objective was to build up Amir's legs. As with all sports, your legs are your foundation. If you get hit, sometimes the strength of your legs is the only thing keeping you from hitting the canvas. Alex's job was to redistribute that muscle up top to Amir's legs. My job was to make sure Amir was getting enough nutrients in the right ratios so that in combination with the training, he would be able to build that muscle in his legs and still lose from his upper body. Too many calories and/or too much protein would result in his building lower body muscle, but he would maintain upper body size. Too few calories and/or too little protein and he would lose upper body size but be unable to bulk up his legs. As always, you need the proper balance of nutrients in conjunction with a systematic training program.

The other major concern was that as Amir had gained upper body mass, it had become more and more difficult for him to make weight. He had been doing crazy cardio to make weight all the way up until the day before his fights. While his body fat percentage was extremely low, all that muscle was working against him.

(Photo: Kazumichi)

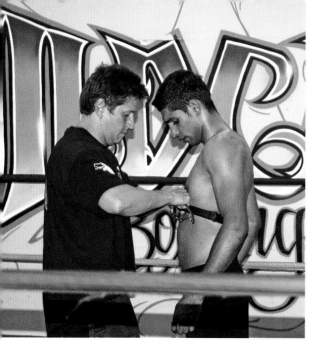
Amir Khan wearing a heart monitor to help pinpoint his metabolic rate.

As with all my clients, the first thing we did was to determine how many calories Amir was burning at rest and in exercise. I placed him on the Body-Gem® to find out what his resting metabolic rate is—about 1880 calories. Amir then wore a heart rate monitor for all of his cardio and strength and conditioning sessions. He started out burning a whopping 1233 calories a day, and that number would progressively increase as his training volume and intensity increased. His basic plan shook out to about 3800 calories.

Another thing we did right off the bat was to simplify Amir's supplement regimen. He first arrived in LA with about a half dozen supplements including creatine, branched chain amino acids, glutamine, a vegetable drink, magnesium, and fish oil. We decided to wipe the slate clean and start out with just a basic high-quality vitamin/mineral supplement and an omega-3 capsule. My feeling is that at this elite level, the bulk of the work is in your foundation—your workouts and your diet. The rest is just icing on the cake. As I've said elsewhere in this book, a good vitamin/mineral acts as insurance against cumulative depletion of nutrients due to topsoil deficiencies, pollutants, and oxidation caused by exercise. I also like fish oil for its anti-inflammatory properties.

But other than those two, while other supplements taken at correct dosages may not hurt you, they may not help you either. Also, in the event that something isn't working, it's harder to pinpoint the source of the problem. And in Amir's case, I really think the creatine, and its subsequent water retention, was making it even harder for him to make weight. The week before the fight, by the way, I had a chance to talk with Amir's physician, who is also the physician for the Premier League's Bolton Wanderers. We were on the same page in our back-to-basics approach to supplements.

Over the next 6 weeks we could see Amir's body changing before our eyes. He had lost much of that muscle from his back and had bulked up his legs. His punches were even faster than they'd been before he came to LA. And he'd regained that footwork and movement that had made him so good as an amateur. The week of the fight, he was down 3.88 pounds in muscle and 2.12 pounds in fat.

Amir Khan: Body Comp Chart

BODY FAT PERCENTAGE TRACKING

	INITIAL	FOLLOW UP 6	CHANGE Since Initial Assessment
NAME: Amir			
WEIGHT:	145.00 lbs	139.00 lbs	-6.00 lbs
LEAN BODY MASS:	137.78 lbs	133.90 lbs	-3.88 lbs
FAT BODY MASS:	7.22 lbs	5.10 lbs	-2.12 lbs
BODY FAT PERCENTAGE:	4.98 %	3.67 %	-1.31 %

teri TOM

Method: Jackson-Pollock   Sum of 7

Follow Up	DATE (mm/dd/yy)	WEIGHT (lbs)	TRICEPS	ILLIAC CREST	THIGH	CHEST	ABDOMEN	SUBSCAPULA	AXILA	Body Fat %	Lean Mass	Fat Mass	BF %	Weight	Lean Mass	Fat Mass
					SITES								Changes since LAST Follow Up			
0	10/20/08	145.00	5.00	4.50	8.00	5.25	7.50	7.00	6.50	4.98%	137.78 lbs	7.22 lbs	0.00%	0.00 lbs	0.00 lbs	0.00 lbs
1	10/27/08	145.50	6.00	5.50	4.75	4.50	6.00	7.50	4.00	4.08%	139.56 lbs	5.94 lbs	-0.89%	0.50 lbs	1.78 lbs	-1.28 lbs
2	11/03/08	144.00	5.50	5.50	5.00	4.50	6.25	7.00	4.00	4.00%	138.24 lbs	5.76 lbs	-0.08%	-1.50 lbs	-1.32 lbs	-0.18 lbs
3	11/10/08	144.00	5.50	6.00	7.00	4.00	6.00	7.50	4.00	4.37%	137.71 lbs	6.29 lbs	0.37%	0.00 lbs	-0.53 lbs	0.53 lbs
4	11/17/08	143.00	5.50	5.00	6.75	4.00	6.50	7.00	4.00	4.16%	137.05 lbs	5.95 lbs	-0.20%	-1.00 lbs	-0.66 lbs	-0.34 lbs
5	11/26/08	140.00	5.00	4.50	7.00	3.50	5.50	7.00	4.00	3.79%	134.69 lbs	5.31 lbs	-0.37%	-3.00 lbs	-2.36 lbs	-0.64 lbs
6	12/03/08	139.00	6.00	5.00	5.00	3.50	5.00	7.00	3.50	3.67%	133.90 lbs	5.10 lbs	-0.13%	-1.00 lbs	-0.79 lbs	-0.21 lbs

End of records

In the weeks leading up to the fight, you can see he gradually dropped weight from 145 to 143 in week four. We started to taper two weeks before the fight, taking out the evening protein snack. When he hit 140, it was my job to keep him there until just a few days before the fight on December 7th. We checked his weight everyday, once in the morning and once after his afternoon workout. Depending on where he was, we'd increase or decrease a snack or two, usually in 100–200 calorie increments, to keep him at 140.

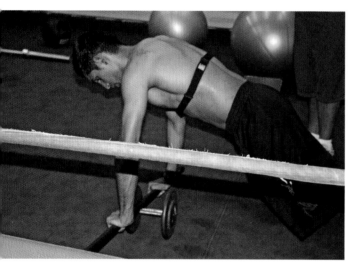

Stabilization exercises are an important part of Amir Khan's supplemental training.

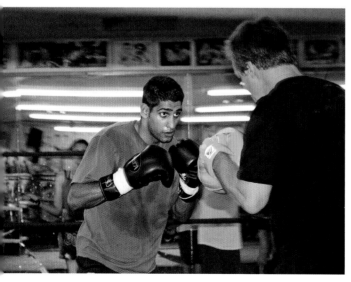

Amir works the mitts with Freddie Roach.

We also played with the ratios, decreasing some of the protein and increasing fat intake. This seemed to do the trick. Alex had laid the foundation in the 5 weeks before we left for London, so Amir's metabolism was firing on all cylinders. By altering these nutrient ratios, then, Amir would lose some of the muscle—and weight—but not strength. On December 3rd, 4 days before the fight, we started to taper more aggressively, removing the morning, afternoon, and evening snacks, and halving the mid-morning snack. On the 4th, he was down to 138. On the 5th, 137. And on the 6th, 136. For the weigh in, he was 135 on the dot.

Later, his manager told us that this was the most relaxed he'd ever seen Amir while making weight. And most important, he didn't have to kill himself this time around. We continued to taper his workouts to the minimum that would allow him to stay sharp, and the night before the weigh-in, he only did some light cardio. A far cry from having to run miles and miles the week of a fight.

The best part of course, was that Amir came back with a spectacular 2nd round knockout victory that should put a stop to all those who had doubted him just a few months earlier.

Amir Khan: Caloric Template

Time	Food	Amount	Grams			
			Cals	Carb	Pro	Fat
6:00	graham crackers	1 ½ sheets	119.5	22	4.5	1.5
	Protein 2 Go	1 pack	52.5	2	10	0.5
8:30	oatmeal	½ c uncooked	162	30	6	2
	milk	8 oz	89	12	8	1
	Designer Whey	2 scoops	204	6	36	4
	berries	1 c	60	15	0	0
	flax seed oil	2 teaspoons	81	0	0	9
11:00	toast	2 slices	162	30	6	2
	chicken, turkey, fish, beef	6 oz cooked	190.5	0	42	2.5
	olive oil	2 teaspoons	90	0	0	10
	butter	2 pats	90	0	0	10
	unlimited veggies		0			
2:00	fruit	1 piece or 1 cup	60	15	0	0
	Protein 2 Go	1 pack	52.5	2	10	0.5
	olives (or 12 nuts)	16 large	90	0	0	10
4:00	Gatorade	32 oz	224	56	0	0
5:00	oatmeal	½ c uncooked	162	30	6	2
	milk	8 oz	89	12	8	1
	Designer Whey	2 scoops	204	6	36	4
	berries	1 c	60	15	0	0
	almonds, pistachios, cashews	12 nuts	90	0	0	10
	flax seed oil	2 teaspoons	81	0	0	9
	olives (or 12 nuts)	16 large	90	0	0	10
7:00	rice	2 c cooked	486	90	18	6
	chicken, turkey, fish, beef	9 oz cooked	495	0	63	27
	oil in cooking	3 tsp approx	135	0	0	15
	unlimited veggies		0			
9:30	milk	8 oz	89	12	8	1
	Designer Whey	1 scoop	102	3	18	2
		Grams Total		358.00	279.50	140.00
		Caloric Total	3810.00	1432.00	1118.00	1260.00

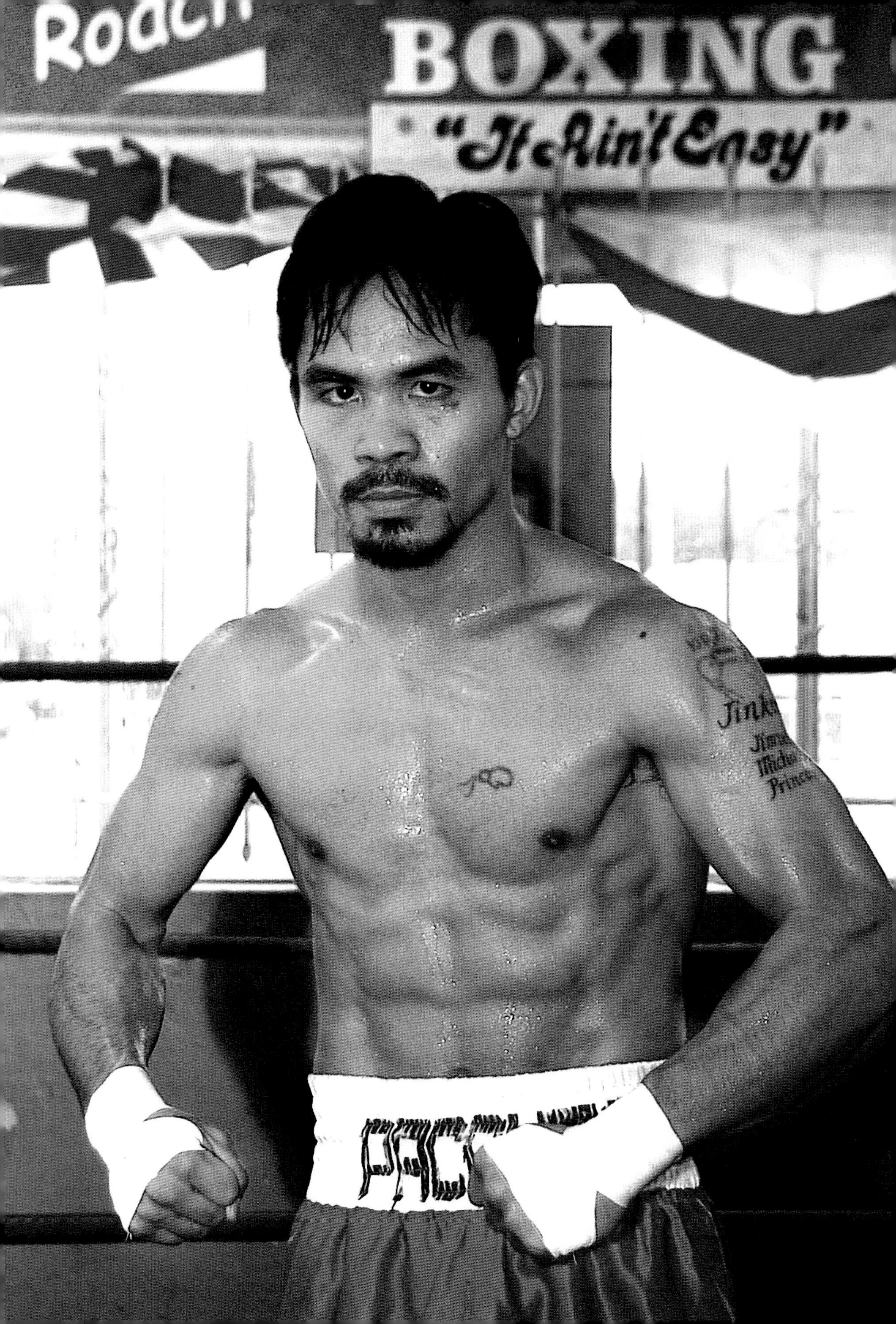

Manny Pacquiao

I started working with Manny Pacquiao in 2008 in preparation for his fight with Oscar De La Hoya. Because Pacquiao would be moving up a whopping two weight classes to meet De La Hoya at 147 pounds, trainer Freddie Roach and conditioning coach Alex Ariza thought it would be a good idea to empirically track Manny's body composition and then make dietary adjustments as needed. After all, Manny would be fighting a naturally bigger man, with a 3-inch reach advantage and 3-and-a-half-inch height advantage.

The main emphasis was on preserving as much muscle as possible. Manny has a history of dipping into the 130s only several weeks into training, which was fine when he was fighting at a lower weight, but this time we had to keep him heavy so he'd have some heft going into the ring with Oscar.

On September 19, 2008, we did a preliminary weigh in before Manny took off for a press tour to promote the fight. At 153, he was only 6.32% body fat which led me to believe that in his previous fights he had made weight by losing a ton of muscle. This time around, we'd have to hold on to as much of that muscle as possible.

The first thing we did was to increase the frequency of meals so as to have shorter intervals between them. For all of his

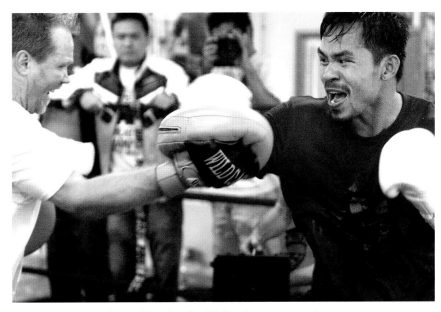

Manny Pacquiao practicing with trainer Freddie Roach. *(Photo: Kazumichi)*

previous fights, Manny had only been eating three times a day with dinner sometimes being as late as 5, 6, or 7 hours after lunch. He was also doing his morning roadwork on an empty stomach, which is fine when you need to shed muscle and weight, but we were trying to keep his weight up.

The other initial change we made was switching his supplements. I won't name names but for years he had been taking a popular multi-vitamin/mineral that did

Manny Pacquiao: Body Comp Chart

BODY FAT PERCENTAGE TRACKING

© 2000-2006 Lucho Crisalle, RD

NAME: Manny

	INITIAL	FOLLOW UP 7	CHANGE Since Initial Assessment
WEIGHT:	153.00 lbs	149.80 lbs	-3.20 lbs
LEAN BODY MASS:	143.32 lbs	142.68 lbs	-0.65 lbs
FAT BODY MASS:	9.68 lbs	7.12 lbs	-2.55 lbs
BODY FAT PERCENTAGE:	6.32 %	4.76 %	-1.57 %

Method: Jackson-Pollock   Sum of 7

Follow Up	DATE (mm/dd/yy)	WEIGHT (lbs)	TRICEPS	ILLIAC CREST	THIGH	CHEST	ABDOMEN	SUBSCAPULA	AXILA	Body Fat %	Lean Mass	Fat Mass	BF %	Weight	Lean Mass	Fat Mass
0	09/19/08	153.00	5.00	7.00	6.50	4.60	9.00	9.00	5.00	6.32%	143.32 lbs	9.68 lbs	0.00%	0.00 lbs	0.00 lbs	0.00 lbs
1	10/06/08	150.00	5.00	7.25	6.00	5.14	9.50	7.75	5.00	6.25%	140.63 lbs	9.37 lbs	-0.07%	-3.00 lbs	-2.70 lbs	-0.30 lbs
2	10/13/08	153.00	6.00	7.50	6.50	5.50	8.50	7.50	5.00	6.39%	143.23 lbs	9.77 lbs	0.14%	3.00 lbs	2.60 lbs	0.40 lbs
3	10/20/08	151.00	5.00	6.00	5.50	4.00	7.50	7.00	5.00	5.33%	142.95 lbs	8.05 lbs	-1.06%	-2.00 lbs	-0.28 lbs	-1.72 lbs
4	10/27/08	153.00	5.00	4.00	5.25	4.50	6.00	7.00	4.50	4.71%	145.79 lbs	7.21 lbs	-0.62%	2.00 lbs	2.84 lbs	-0.84 lbs
5	11/03/08	152.00	5.00	5.00	5.00	4.00	6.00	7.00	4.50	4.76%	144.77 lbs	7.23 lbs	0.04%	-1.00 lbs	-1.02 lbs	0.02 lbs
6	11/10/08	151.00	5.00	4.00	5.50	3.75	5.00	6.50	4.00	4.30%	144.51 lbs	6.49 lbs	-0.45%	-1.00 lbs	-0.27 lbs	-0.73 lbs
7	11/17/08	149.80	5.00	4.50	5.50	4.50	6.00	7.00	4.00	4.76%	142.68 lbs	7.12 lbs	0.45%	-1.20 lbs	-1.83 lbs	0.63 lbs

End of records

not rate well with third-party research. True, he'd gone pretty far on that supplement, but he was going to need every edge possible for this fight. To convince him to make a switch, I ran a little experiment and placed apple slices in water with different supplements. When apples are exposed to oxygen, they turn brown—hence, the word oxidation. A high quality vitamin-mineral should protect the apple from browning, which ours did, well after several days. The apple was actually its natural color and I was able to bite into it. The apple soaked in the supplement that Manny had been taking turned black. Not brown.

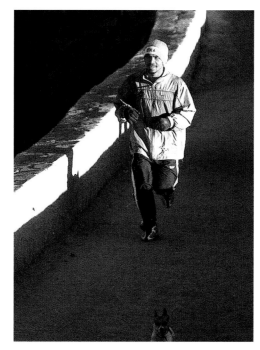

Manny used a morning run as part of his conditioning regimen. *(Photo: Kazumichi)*

Black. The apple slice in plain water turned brown and looked a heckuva lot better than the black one. Which probably backs up my opinion that you're better off not doing any supplements instead of a bad one. In any case, Manny started taking the high quality multi-vit/mineral to help with post-workout recovery.

We started making dietary adjustments just after he returned from the press tour. You can see during a week of inactivity, he'd already lost 2.7 pounds of muscle and 0.3 pounds fat. From there we introduced the protein shake in the morning, about 20 grams, before his run and another 20 grams after his afternoon workout. This in combination with his strength and conditioning sessions with Alex enabled him to regain any lost ground the next week, and he climbed right back up to 153.

During the third week, he dipped a little bit in muscle, so we started giving him a mid-morning snack as well—usually an egg sandwich—right after his morning run. He popped up 2.84 pounds in muscle.

It's important to remember that the volume and intensity of Manny's workouts were progressively increasing during training camp. This is why we had to make constant adjustments. With each week, he would be running more sets of sprints, sparring more rounds, and doing more strength and conditioning circuits. So in week five, he dipped again in muscle. At this point, he was eating enough times during the day, but he was not eating enough protein at his larger meals. When I would have lunch or dinner with him, I would simply point to protein dishes and remind him to have more. Usually, he would try to get *me* to eat more with him!

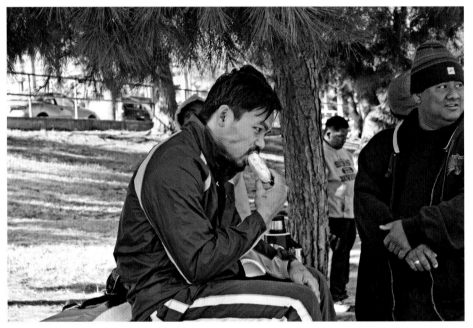

The timing and amounts of nutrients are key, especially during an intense training program. Here, Manny Pacquiao eats an egg sandwich after his morning run.

This is where I should mention the Thai restaurant. If you watch HBO's *24/7*, you know he likes to eat there after every workout. I am asked all the time, "What do you think about the Thai restaurant?" Like it's some horrible thing. Frankly, when you're Manny Pacquiao, you burn through calories like there's no tomorrow. My feeling is if he's 4–6% body fat and losing muscle is a concern, I am not going to quibble about the Thai restaurant and coconut sauces. It's more important that he get those calories in and that it's palatable to him and that he enjoys his food, because he really needs it. A lot of people ask me about the four cups of rice he'll have. Again, not a problem when body fat is coming down and we are preserving muscle. So in the sixth week, I just asked that he eat a little more protein at lunch and dinner and the next week he only dropped a quarter of a pound in muscle, which was not too big of a deal since we would gradually have to come down to 147 anyway.

Then in the seventh week, he dropped almost two pounds in muscle all the way down to 149.8, which was much too fast of a drop. We were still three weeks away from tapering his training and diet leading up to the fight. I asked him what happened. For some odd reason, he'd forgotten to take the protein shakes in the mornings that week. Hey, it happens to all of us—sometimes you just go off the rails a bit even if it's unintentional. But combined with his increased exercise load, he was losing muscle too fast. You'll also see that he gained 0.63 pounds in fat, which means he wasn't getting enough calories, let alone protein.

Unfortunately, this is where I had to leave LA to travel to London with Amir Khan in preparation for Amir's fight (on the same night, if you can believe it!). So it was up to Alex to get Manny back on track for the fight, which he did. They went back to the original plan, with Alex increasing protein and meal frequency at every opportunity— before the morning run, mid-morning, after the afternoon workout, and before bed. This seemed to turn things around, and despite the official weigh-in results, according to the scales at the hotel, Manny left for the weigh-in at 146.5.

Not that it really matters, does it? With the odds stacked against him, Manny had more than enough weight behind his punches to score the upset of his career, beating De La Hoya in the eighth round.

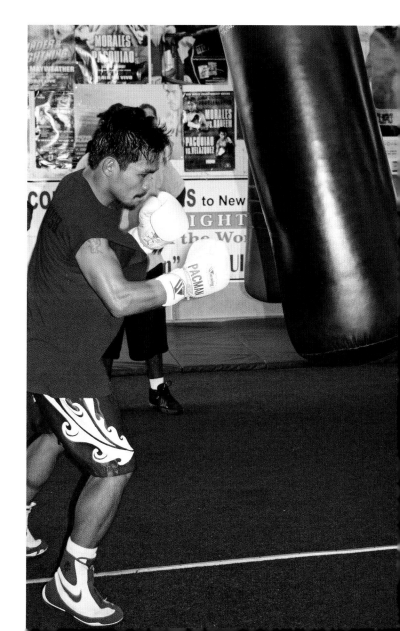

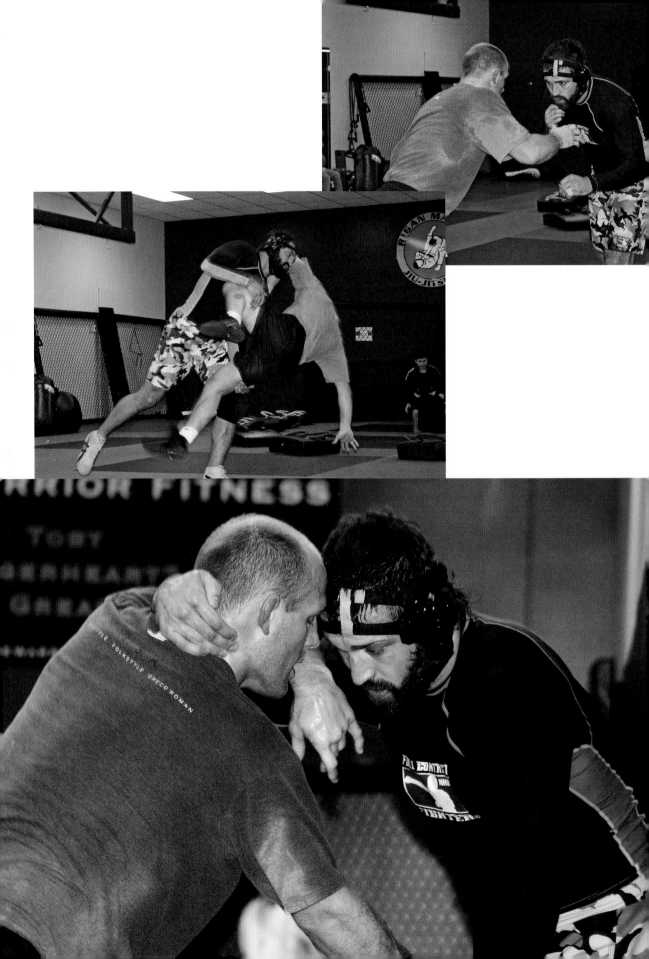

Andrei Arlovski

When I was first asked to work with Andrei Arlovski, our main concern was his conditioning. He was about to embark on a pro boxing career but at the same time was still competing in MMA. This presented unique nutrition challenges because he was training three times a day in three different modes—conditioning, boxing, and grappling. His coach Freddie Roach was concerned that Andrei might gas out in the latter rounds of a fight.

As is always my philosophy, "if it ain't broke, don't fix it." There weren't major changes to make to Andrei's diet. And just as was the case with Pacquiao's nutrition plan, I don't believe in changing a fighter's diet too drastically if it can be helped. I've heard horror stories of nutritionists who tried to impose diets that are too rigid, too low in fat, too low in carbs, or just too exotic. I've seen such diets implemented too close to fights with disastrous results. If ostrich meat is something not usually in a fighter's diet, then I would avoid it altogether.

Much in the same way people ask me if I approve of Pacquiao's frequenting the Thai restaurant, I was once asked at an Italian restaurant about the three entrees Andrei ordered. I said if he needs the calories—which he clearly does not only because of the volume of his training schedule, but also because of the sheer amount of muscle mass he has to support—and if he enjoys the food, by all means order three entrees of Italian food!

In fact, getting Andrei to consume more food at more frequent intervals was our main modification. The tendency was for his body fat percentage to dip too low, and this seemed to correspond to fatigue in the ring and in the latter weeks of training camp. We encouraged him to take in more fat. We also introduced protein shakes supplemented with flax seed oil at mid-morning and mid-afternoon. The mid-afternoon snack was crucial, since he would be going from sparring in the ring straight to a grappling session. He would often not get to dinner until 8 o'clock at night, so an adequate meal prior to the session was necessary to maintain muscle mass and keep body fat up. As always, weekly monitoring gave us the information we needed to know what direction to take.

Remember, there is always a trade-off between composition and performance. What's good for a magazine cover isn't necessarily the best thing for a fight. You can always regain your six-pack afterwards, but it's better to have some reserves to tap into during the actual fight.

Parting Shots

Based on the information in this book, you can see why I insist on your being methodical in your approach to fitness. You need to have your bases covered on all three—nutrition, exercise, and mental—fronts. Without a sound plan for any of these three components, you won't be able to break through those plateaus when you hit them.

But by tracking both food portions and ratios, by knowing the specific parameters of your exercise, by monitoring your progress regularly and knowing how to take action based on that knowledge, and, most important, by tapping into your own motivations for following a program in the first place—by not leaving anything to chance, you have no alternative but to succeed. You'll also reach your goals as efficiently as possible, because you'll be able to detect plateaus and undesirable results immediately—and you'll know how to correct them.

The other thing to remember is that you are in this for the long haul. As I've said before, an all-or-nothing approach can be detrimental in the long run. If you have a bad day, don't use it as an excuse to scrap the whole week. Just get back in that saddle. As you've seen from the client examples provided here, one bad result doesn't sabotage the entire project. A lot of my clients say their charts look like the stock market—as long as the overall trend is in the desired direction, we're okay. Think Big Picture, because this is not a diet or a temporary plan.

Because our bodies are *always* changing—yes, even as you're reading this—give yourself an acceptable body fat *range,* and not a fixed number, that you'll want to maintain. This allows you to pop up slightly or have a bad day or two, but keeps you always within striking distance. If you have a fight or an event for which you want to lean out and/or bulk up, you won't have too much work to do. Constantly yo-yoing between extremes is both psychologically draining and physically taxing. Even worse, the more yo-yoing you do, the less your body will respond the next time. Consistency and moderation are key.

I've given you all the tools you'll need. It's time for me to pass the torch. It's up to you now. Whether you're a professional fighter, serious martial artist, elite athlete, weekend warrior, or someone starting out on the fitness path for the first time, follow the steps as I've outlined them here, and your efforts will be a surefire success. For additional information, please visit my website at www. teritom.com. I look forward to hearing all of your success stories!

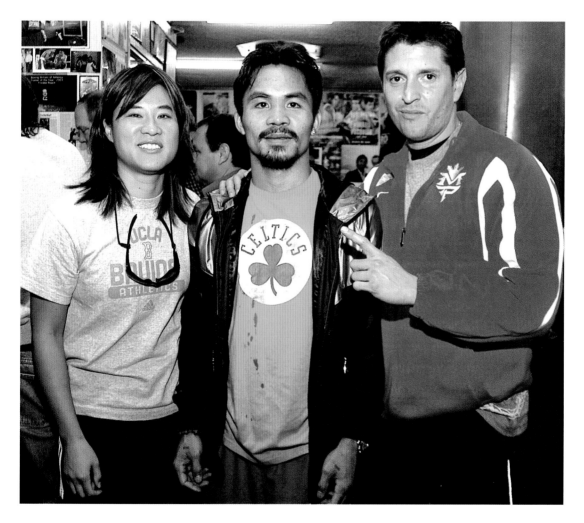

Teri Tom posing with client Manny Pacquiao and conditioning coach Alex Ariza. *(Photo: Kazumichi)*

HOW TO FIND A REGISTERED DIETITIAN

We've covered a lot of information in this book. You may want to seek some outside advisement to add to your knowledge or to get you started properly. But where do you start?

Anytime you seek advice or information you want to be sure it comes from a qualified source—especially when that advice pertains to your body and your health. Remember the commercial that begins with "I'm not a doctor, but I play one on TV." Well, would you trust an actor to operate on you? I didn't think so. The same should go for nutrition advice. Unfortunately, in some states anyone can call himself or herself a "nutritionist," and that includes actors. And did you know that even doctors often only receive 1 to 5 days of nutrition education in med school?

So who's the Go-To Guy or Gal when it comes to nutrition advice? You should look for someone sporting the initials "RD" after his or her name. The "RD" stands for Registered Dietitian, which means that person has completed the necessary requirements determined by the Commission on Dietetic Registration (CDR). This is the credentialing agency for the American Dietetic Association (ADA). The requirements to become a Registered Dietitian include completion of core curriculum in a nutrition related four-year college degree from an accredited university, completion of a yearlong (or more) internship, and passing the CDR's registration exam. To maintain their license, RD's must also complete continuing education courses.

And as we mentioned in one of the case studies, if you're active, you'll want to find a dietitian who knows how to incorporate your exercise routine into your nutrition plan. Look for dietitians with additional degrees or certifications in personal training and exercise physiology.

Other Reliable Resources

If you're hunting for sound nutrition information on the Internet, beware. There's a whole universe of commercial websites dying to sell you their products. And they'll use so-called "third-party" studies to support their claims. Don't be fooled. Instead, try these websites, many of which include peer-reviewed journals.

MEDLINE database
www.nlm.nih.gov/medlineplus/

ConsumerLab
www.consumerlab.com

The American Journal of Clinical Nutrition
www.ajcn.org

Supplement Watch
www.supplementwatch.com

Food and Drug Administration
www.cfsan.fda.gv

Institute of Food Technologies
www.ift.org

National Institutes of Health, Office of Dietary Supplements
www.ods.od.nih.gov

NOTES

1. Morihei Ueshiba, *The Secret Teachings of Aikido* (Tokyo: Kodansha, 2007), p. 30.

2. Daisets T. Suzuki, *Zen and Japanese Culture* (Princeton: Princeton University Press, 1959), p. 99.

3. Bruce Lee, ed. John Little, *Jeet Kune Do: Bruce Lee's Commentaries on the Martial Way* (Boston: Tuttle Publishing, 1997), p. 353.

4. Omori Sogen, *An Introduction to Zen Training* (North Clarendon, Vt.: Tuttle Publishing, 1996), p. 130.

5. Suzuki, *Zen and Japanese Culture*, p. 101.

6. Ibid., p. 62.

7. Ibid., p. 142.

8. Ibid., p. 72.

9. Sogen, *An Introduction to Zen Training*, p. 130.

10. Bruce Lee, ed. John Little, *Bruce Lee: The Art of Expressing the Human Body* (North Clarendon, Vt.: Tuttle Publishing, 1998), p. 162.

11. Sogen, *An Introduction to Zen Training*, p. 6.

12. Kenji Tokitsu, *Miyamoto Musashi: His Life and Writings* (Boston: Weatherhill, 2004), p. 287.

13. Suzuki, *Zen and Japanese Culture*, p. 157.

14. *Brit. J. Sports Med.* 2003 Jun: 37(3):245–9.

15. Coyle EF, Hagberg JM, Hurley BF, et al. Carbohydrate feeding during prolonged strenuous exercise can delay fatigue. *J. Appl. Physiology.* 1983; 55(1 Pt 1):230–235.

16. Saunders MJ, Kane MD, Todd MK. Effects of carbohydrate-protein beverage on cycling endurance and muscle damage. *Med. Sci. Sports Exercise.* 2004; 36(7):1233–1238.

17. Van Essen M, Gibala MJ. Failure of protein to improve time trial performance when added to a sports drink. *Med. Sci. Sports Exercise.* 2006; 38(8):1476–1483.

18. Jackson AS, and Pollock ML: Generalized equations for predicting body density of women. *Med. Sci. Sports,* 12:175, 1980.

19. Jackson AS, and Pollock ML: Generalized equations for predicting body density of men. *Brit. J. Nutr.,* 40:497, 1978.

20. Heyward VH, and Stolarczyk LM: *Applied Body Composition Assessment.* Champaign, IL: Human Kinetics, 1996.

21. Filaire E, Maso F, Degoutte F, Jouanel P, Lac G, Food restriction, performance, psychological state and lipid values in judo athletes. *Int. J. Sports Med.* 2001 Aug; 22(6):454–9.

22. Hall CJ, Lane AM, Effects of rapid weight loss on mood and performance among amateur boxers. *Br J Sports Med.* 2001 Dec; 35(6):390–5.

23. Phillips T, Childs AC, Dreon DM, et al. A dietary supplement attenuates IL-6 and CRP after eccentric exercise in untrained males. *Med Sci Sports Exercise.* 2003; 35(12):2032–2037.

24. Calder PC. n-3 polyunsaturated fatty acids, inflammation, and inflammatory diseases. *Am J Clin Nutr.* 2006; 83(6): S1505–1519S.

25. Van Somere KA, Edwards AJ, Howatson G. Supplementation with beta-hydroxy-beta-methylbutyrate (HMB) and alpha-ketoiscaproic acid (KIC) reduces signs and symptoms of exercise-induced muscle damage in man. *Int. J. Sport Nutr. Exerc. Metab.* 2005; 15(4):413–424.

26. Coombes JS, McNaughton LR. Effects of branched-chain amino acid supplementation on serum creatine kinase and lactate dehydrogenase after prolonged exercise. *J. Sports Med. Phys. Fitness.* 2000, 40(3):240–246.

27. Kreider RB. Effects of creatine supplementation on performance and training adaptations. *Mol. Cell. Biochem.* 2003; 244(1–2):89–94.

28. Santos RV, Bassit RA, Caperuto EC, et al. The effect of creatine supplementation upon inflammatory and muscle soreness markers after a 30 km race. *Life Sci.* 2004; 75(16): 1917–1924.

29. Favano A, Santos-Silva PR, Nakano EY, Pedrinelli A, Hernandez A.J, Greve JM. Peptide glutamine supplentation for tolerance of intermittent exercise in soccer players. *Clinics*, 2008 Feb; 63(1):27–32.

30. Bassini-Cameron A, Monteiro A, Gomes A, Werneck-de-Castro JP, Cameron L. Glutamine protects against increases in blood ammonia in football players in an exercise intensity-dependent way. *Brit. J. Sports Med.* 2008 Apr; 42(4): 260–6.

31. Herrero-Beaumont G, Ivorra JA, Del Carmen Trabado M, Blanco FJ, Benito P, Martin-Mola E, Paulino J, Marcenco JL, Porto A, Laffon A, Araujo D, Figueroa M, Branco J. Glucosamine sulfate in the treatment of knee osteoarthritis symptoms: a randomized, double-blind, placebo-controlled study using acetaminophen as a side comparator. *Arthritis Rheum.* 2007 Feb; 56(2):555–67.

32. Hespel P, Maughan RJ, Greenhaff PL. Dietary supplements for football. *J Sports Sci.* 2006 Jul; 24(7):749–61.

33. Leffler CT, Phillippi AF, Leffler SG, Mosure JC, Kim PD. Glucosamine, chondroitin, and manganese ascorbate for degenerative joint disease of the knee or low back: a randomized, double-blind, placebo-controlled pilot study. *Mil. Med.* 1999 Feb; 164(2): 85–91.

34. For more information about Sensei Freedman, visit his website at *www.freedmansmethod.com*. He specializes in Ketsugo Jujutsu, Arnis, Kali, Escrima, Spirit Training, and Law Enforcement training and teaches seminars, workshops, and private lessons. He can be contacted at his school in Weare, New Hampshire at (603) 529-3564.

REFERENCES

Ainsworth, B.A., Haskell, W.L., Leon, A.S., et al. (1993). Compendium of physical activities: classification of energy costs of human physical activities. *Medicine and Science in Sports and Exercise, 25,* 71–80.

Akermark, C., Jacobs, I., Rasmussinm, M., & Karlson, J. (1996). Diet and muscle glycogen concentration in relation to physical performance in Swedish elite ice hockey players. *International Journal of Sports Nutrition, 6,* 272–284.

American College of Sports Medicine (1996). Position stand: exercise and fluid Replacement. *Medicine and Science in Sports and Exercise, 28,* i–vii.

American Dietetic Association & Canadian Dietetic Association (1993). Nutrition for physical fitness and athletic performance in adults. *Journal of the American Dietetic Association, 93,* 691–696.

Balsom, P.D., Wood, K., Olsson, P., & Ekblom, B. (1999). Carbohydrate intake and multiple sprint sports with special reference to football (soccer). *International Journal of Sports Medicine, 20,* 48–52.

Bernardot, D. (2000). *Nutrition for Serious Athletes.* 1st ed. Champaign: Human Kinetics.

Bishop, N.C., Blannin, A.K., & Glesson, M., et al. (2000). Effect of carbohydrate and fluid intake during prolonged exercise on saliva flow and IGA secretion. *Medicine and Science in Sports and Exercise, 32 (12), 2046–2051.*

Bishop, N.C., Blannin, A.K., Rand, L., et al. (1999). Effects of carbohydrate intake on the blood leukocyte responses to prolonged cycling. *Journal of Sports Science, 17,* 26–7.

Brownell, K.D., Nelson-Steen, S., & Wilmore, J.H. (1987). Weight regulation practices in athletes: analysis of metabolic and health effects. *Medicine and Science in Sports and Exercise, 18,* 546–556.

Butterfield, G. (1991). Amino acids and high protein diets. In Lamb D. & Williams, M. (eds.), *Perspectives in Exercise Science and Sports Medicine* (pp. 87–122). Carmel, IN: Cooper Publishing Group.

Butterfield, G. (1987). Whole-body protein utilization in humans. *Medicine and Science in Sports and Exercise, 19,* S157–65.

Carraro, F., et al. (1990). Effect of exercise and recovery on muscle protein synthesis in human subjects. *American Journal of Physiology, 259,* E470.

Coyle, E.F. & Montain, S.J. (1992). Benefits of fluid replacement with carbohydrate during exercise. *Medicine and Science in Sports and Exercise, 24,* S324–330.

Craig, B.W. (1993). The influence of fructose feeding on physical performance. *American Journal of Clinical Nutrition, 58,* S815.

Davis, J.M., Burgess, W.A., Slents, C.A., Bartoli, W.P., & Pate, R.R. (1988). Effects of ingesting 6% and 12% glucose-electrolyte beverages during prolonged intermittent cycling in the heat. *European Journal of Applied Physiology, 57,* 563–569.

Davy, B. (2000). Managing body weight. In C.A. Rosenbloom (ed.), *Sports nutrition: a guide for the professional working with active people* (pp. 430–431). Chicago: The American Dietetic Association.

Duyff, R.L. (2002). *American Dietetic Association food and nutrition guide* (2nd ed.). Chicago: The American Dietetic Association.

Eicher, E.R., Mahan, J., Painter, P., & Zambraski, E. (1994). Roundtable: the kidney, exercise, and hydration. *Sports Science Exchange, 5* (3).

Fleck, S.J. (1983). Body composition of elite American athletes. *American Journal of Sports Medicine, 11,* 398–403.

Foster-Powel, K., & Miller, J.R. (1995). International tables of glycemic index. *American Journal of Clinical Nutrition, 62,* 871S–93S.

Hickson, J.F., et al. (1990). Repeated days of body building exercise do not enahnce urinary nitrogen excretions from untrained young males. *Nutrition Research, 10,* 723.

Houtkooper, L. B., Going, S.B. (1994). Body composition: how should it be measured? Does it affect performance? *Sports Science Exchange, 7* (5).

Hubbard, R.W., Szlyk, P.C., & Armstrong, L.E. (1990). Influence of thirst and fluid palatibility on fluid ingestion during exercise. In Gisulfi, C.V., & Lamg, D.R. (eds.), *Fluid homeostasis during exercise* (pp. 39–95). Carmel, IN: Benchmark Press.

Kurtzweil, P. An FDA guide to dietary supplements. (1998, September-October). *FDA Consumer Magazine.* Retrieved December 13, 1998 from http://www.fdagov/fdac/features/1998/598-guid.html

Langly, S. (2000). Managing body weight. In C.A. Rosenbloom (ed.), *Sports nutrition: a guide for the professional working with active people* (pp. 587–597). Chicago: The American Dietetic Association.

Lemon, P.W. (1996). Is increased dietary protein necessary or beneficial for individuals with a physically active lifestyle? *Nutrition Review, 54,* S169–75.

Lightsey, D., & Attaway, J. (1992). Deceptive tactics used in marketing purported ergogenic aids. *National Strength and Conditioning Association Journal, 14,* 14:26–31.

Little, J. (1998). *The art of expressing the human body.* Boston: Tuttle Publishing.

Little, J. (1997). *Jeet kune do: Bruce Lee's commentaries on the martial way.* Boston: Tuttle Publishing.

Maughaun, R.J., & Leiper, J.B. (1994). Fluid requirements in soccer. *Journal of Sports Science, 12,* S29.

McArdle, W.D., Katch, F.L., & Katch, V.L. (1999). *Sports and exercise nutrition.* Baltimore: Lippincott, Williams, & Wilkins.

Meridith, C.N., et al. (1989). Dietary protein requirements and body protein metabolism in endurance-trained men. *Journal of Applied Physiology, 66,* 2580.

Murray, R., Paul, G.L., Seifert, J.G., Eddy, D.E., & Halaby, G.A. (1989). The effects of glucose, fructose, and sucrose ingestion during exercise. *Medicine and Science in Sports and Exercise, 21,* 275–282.

Norwalk, R.K., Knudsen, K.S., & Schulz, L.O. (1988). Body composition and nutrient intakes of college men and women basketball players. *Journal of the American Dietetic Association, 88,* 575–578.

Otis, C., Goldingay, R. (2000). *The Athletic Woman's Survival Guide.* Champaign: Human Kinetics.

Rankin, J.W., Ocel, J.V., & Craft, L.L. (1996). Effect of weight loss and refeeding diet composition on anaerobic performance in wrestlers. *Medicine and Science in Sports and Exercise. 28,* 1292–1299.

Rosa, A.M., & Shizgal, H.M. (1984). The Harris-Benedict equation reevaluated: resting energy requirements and body cell mass. *American Journal of Clinical Nutrition, 40,* 168–182.

Sherman, W.J., & Maglischo, E.W. (1991). Minimizing chronic fatigue among swimmers: special emphasis on nutrition. *Sports Science Exchange, 35* (4).

Shi, X., & Gisuffi, C.V. (1998). Fluid replacement and carbohydrate replacement during intermittent exercise. *Sports Medicine, 25,* 157–172.

Silverman, J. (2002). *The greatest boxing stories ever told.* Guilford, CT: The Lyons Press.

Skov, A.R., Tourbo, S., Ronn, B., Holm, L., & Astrup, A. (1999). Randomized trial on protein vs. carbohydrate in ad libitum fat reduced diet for the treatment of obesity. *International Journal of Obesity Related Metabolic Disorders, 23,* 528–36.

Tarnopolosky, M.A., et al. (1988). Influence of protein intake and training status on nitrogen balance and lean body mass. *Journal of Applied Physiology, 64,* 187.

Tarnopolosky, M.A., et al. (1990). Effect of bodybuilding exercise on protein requirements. *Canadian Journal of Sports Science, 15,* 225.

Vergauwen, L., Brouns, F., & Vespel, P. (1998). Carbohydrate supplementation impoves stroke performance in tennis. *Medicine and Science in Sports and Exercise, 30,* 1289–1295.

Walberg-Rankin, J. (1995). Dietary carbohydrate as an ergogenic aid for prolonged and brief competitions in sport. *International Journal of Sports Nutrition, 5,* S13–S28.

Welsh, R.S., Bryan, S., Bartoli, W., Burke, J.M., Williams, S.H., & Davis, J.M. (1999). Influence of carbohydrate ingestion on physical and mental function during intermittent high-intensity exercise to fatigue. *Medicine and Science in Sports and Exercise, 31,* S123.

Ziegler, P., Nelson J.A., Barratt-Fornell, A., Fiveash, L., & Drewnowski, A. (2001). Energy and macronutrient intakes of elite figure skaters. *Journal of the American Dietetic Association, 101,* 319–325.

INDEX